The Daniel Fast for Weight Loss

Visit Tyndale online at www.tyndale.com.

Visit Tyndale Momentum online at www.tyndalemomentum.com.

Visit the author's website at www.Daniel-Fast.com.

Tyndale Momentum and the Tyndale Momentum logo are registered trademarks of Tyndale House Publishers, Inc. Tyndale Momentum is an imprint of Tyndale House Publishers, Inc.

The Daniel Fast for Weight Loss: A Biblical Approach to Losing Weight and Keeping It Off

Designed by Mark Lane

Published in association with the literary agency of Ann Spangler and Company, 1415 Laurel Ave. SE, Grand Rapids, MI 49506.

Library of Congress Cataloging-in-Publication Data

Gregory, Susan, date.
  The Daniel fast for weight loss : a biblical approach to losing weight and keeping it off / Susan Gregory.
    pages cm
  Includes bibliographical references and index.
  ISBN 978-1-4964-0748-1 (sc)
  1. Fasting—Religious aspects—Christianity. 2. Human body—Religious aspects—Christianity. 3. Weight loss—Religious aspects—Christianity. 4. Daniel (Biblical figure)
  I. Title.
  BV5055.G743 2015
  613.2'5—dc23   2015023364

Printed in the United States of America

21	20	19	18	17	16	15
7	6	5	4	3	2	1

THE
daniel
fast

for weight loss

a biblical approach to losing weight and keeping it off

susan gregory

TYNDALE®
MOMENTUM

An Imprint of
Tyndale House Publishers, Inc.

*To all who struggle with weight and health challenges
yet are willing to fight the good fight of faith to overcome
them and step into the victory that awaits you*

Table of Contents

PART ONE

CHAPTER 1

The Daniel Fast

A Spiritual Fast That Encourages Physical Health

A NEW TREND IS EMERGING IN AMERICA, and this one is pointing us in the right direction. The latest fashion statement is health. We hear about it in magazines, on the news, and online, with new studies and suggestions popping up all the time. Yet in a nation where so many good things are available to us, nearly 70 percent of all Americans suffer from food-created ailments. The most widespread are obesity and overweight, which are key contributors to type 2 diabetes, high cholesterol, high blood pressure, heart disease, poor quality of life, and even premature death. If you're concerned about any of these areas—or even if you feel pretty good about your health but want to improve some habits—then this book is for you.

You are holding in your hand a guide that can start you on a life-changing journey to bring health and wellness to your spirit, your soul, and your body. In the pages of this book,

I will lead you into a faith-driven experience that will foster deeply rooted change. I will show how you can embrace some of the ways of God and, by doing so, cause those areas of your life that may be out of order to come into alignment with the heart of your Lord.

I will also introduce you to proven principles that can put an end to the cravings that disrupt your health goals. I will show you how to make minor changes in your daily habits that can cause dramatic improvements in your health and weight loss. And I will lead you through a twenty-one-day Daniel Fast for Weight Loss that will jump-start you into a lifestyle that is satisfying and safe, and will bring you the joy and freedom you desire.

Before we go any further, let me declare an essential point: This is not a diet book! Diets are temporary; you go on one and then you go off of it. Diets are plans you follow for a short period of time for quick results, and I don't think I need to tell you that they don't usually work. You probably know that from your own personal experience. Later on I'll go into more detail about why the Daniel Fast is effective whereas diets often aren't. But for now, please understand, you are not reading another diet book that you'll try for a while to see if it is the silver bullet to end all your weight-loss woes. Instead, you're reading a book that looks beyond temporary physical changes to lasting spiritual transformation.

You will also be guided to a safe, nutritious eating plan that will result in your dropping unwanted pounds without having to tediously count calories. The Daniel Fast meals are well-balanced and satisfying. As you follow the advice in this book, you will find that cravings disappear and you won't even want to overeat. Therefore, there isn't a need to count or track calories.

I don't think you've picked up this book by mistake. You may have an internal and perhaps even unspoken yearning to drop unwanted pounds. You may want to stop sabotaging yourself by giving in to cravings for foods you know aren't good for you. Perhaps the Lord has nudged you many times to lose weight and get healthy.

The Daniel Fast for Weight Loss can initiate lifelong changes to address all of those problems. You can gain the control you thought was unattainable, and even eliminate anxiety and guilt about poor eating habits. In addition, the Daniel Fast will serve as a foundation for your forever healthy lifestyle. Most important, you will be in a place of joy and thanksgiving as you partner with your Creator in this life-giving process of transformation.

MY FASTING JOURNEY

I started fasting in the early 1990s. I had been a Christian for many years, but I wanted a deeper life with Jesus. At first I used a "normal fast" as my method, which means abstaining from food and drinking only water. My fasts were usually only a few days long.

Then in 2005, my life seemed to be exploding on just about every front. I was mature enough in my Christian walk to know that when life seems to be going off the rails, the best choice is to get on God's path and walk with Him in the Spirit (see Galatians 5:25). In the midst of the turmoil, I wanted to draw nearer to God. I decided to enter an extended time of prayer and fasting using the Daniel Fast as my method.

Our God is always faithful. James 4:8 teaches, "Draw near to God and He will draw near to you." And that's exactly what happened during my twenty-one-day Daniel Fast. I faced difficult circumstances, but I felt as if the Lord had cloaked me in a protective robe that guarded me from the agonizing stress and heartache of betrayal that I would otherwise have suffered. He showered me with His precious love and His priceless grace, and He took my hand and showed me how to walk through the dark valley my earthly life had entered.

During this time I learned the incomparable value of extended prayer and fasting. I also realized that the Daniel Fast is a doable method of fasting for long periods of time. Since it's a partial fast, where some foods are restricted and others allowed, I was able to receive the great benefits of biblical fasting for many weeks. Yet I was also able to attend to my responsibilities without the low energy that would occur if I was only drinking water or juice for multiple weeks.

Then in 2007, like millions of others in the United States and around the world, my life was hit harshly with the economic recession. After many months of trying to survive the downturn in the real estate market, I was forced to close my real estate investing business. I felt as if the financial rug had been pulled out from under me. It was stressful and dark, but as before, I knew that while the world was shaking in the uncertain times, the Lord was my solid rock and my safe refuge. Psalm 18 says:

I will love You, O LORD, my strength.
The LORD is my rock and my fortress and my deliverer;
My God, my strength, in whom I will trust;
My shield and the horn of my salvation, my stronghold.
I will call upon the LORD, who is worthy to be praised;
So shall I be saved from my enemies.

PSALM 18:1-3

In the winter of 2007, after hour upon hour of praying and seeking God and His direction, I heard the Spirit of God speaking to me in my spirit. He said, *Write about the Daniel Fast.*

Receiving an assignment from the Lord to write wasn't intimidating for me. I had spent more than twenty years as a Christian writer and had worked for many well-known ministries as a copywriter. I was, however, wondering how I was supposed to get the message about the Daniel Fast out to the Christian community quickly. January was approaching, and I knew that hundreds of thousands of believers throughout the world started the New Year with extended prayer and fasting, and that the most widely used method of fasting was the Daniel Fast. Even I was planning to use the Daniel Fast at the beginning of the coming year.

I was comfortable with computers since I had been a writer and a business owner, but I had never created a website and had no idea what to do. Still, I knew that the fastest way to share information with the most people would be through the Internet. So I put my head down, learned how to create a simple but usable website, and wrote about the Daniel Fast.

To say I was shocked by the response from the public would be a gross understatement. I was genuinely amazed when tens of thousands of people visited my simple website and wanted to learn more. With the rush of visitors and the unexpected popularity of the site, I felt as if I were on a wild amusement-park ride. I worked from dawn until late into the night answering posts and creating helpful tools for my readers, including two e-books. (This was before Kindle and Nook.)

I answered thousands of questions that people posted on the site. If I didn't know the answer to an inquiry, I would research until I could give a biblically based response. And through the hours and hours of writing and researching, I learned the ins and outs of spiritual fasting in general and, more specifically, the Daniel Fast. While I called myself "the Daniel Fast Blogger," I soon become known as "the Daniel Fast Expert."

One of the unforeseen benefits of writing about the Daniel Fast is that I received hundreds and hundreds of testimonies from women and men who had used the fast. The accounts were inspiring to read. God displayed His greatness as He ministered to His children while they fasted. Just about everyone experienced a deepened relationship with the Lord and developed new habits of prayer, meditation, and study. Some received supernatural answers to their prayers, including financial breakthroughs and a path for future stewardship and security. Failing marriages were restored, babies were conceived even after fertility doctors had given no hope, jobs were secured following months of unemployment, and forgiveness was imparted after deep and painful betrayal. One of the most touching testimonies was from a woman who had been estranged from her son for seventeen years. She prayed and asked God to minister to her son's heart, and while she was on the Daniel Fast he called and asked if they could rebuild their relationship.

Among all these powerful testimonies were many that had to do with improved health. While people entered into the fast for the spiritual experience of drawing nearer to God, they were astonished by the improvements in their physical health. People who had high cholesterol before the fast learned that their counts had dropped to safe levels. Men and women with type 2 diabetes were able to drastically reduce or eliminate their body's need for medication; instead, their blood-sugar levels were now controlled by food. Many with high blood pressure reported that they were now in the safe zone, to the surprise of their doctors.

Weight loss was another common report. Without even trying, both men and women on the fast dropped a significant number of pounds. Some shed seven or eight pounds, while a few lost as many as twenty-five. The average loss over the twenty-one-day fasting experience was nine to ten pounds, and this was not because people were starving themselves. Rather, it was because they focused more of their attention on the Lord; ate simple, nourishing meals; and drank only water. A typical comment was, "I haven't felt this good in twenty years. I want to live this way forever!"

Many wanted to know if they could fast as a way of life. However, God designed fasting to last for a short period. It's a tool to help us focus on Him for a specific need or purpose.

What these women and men wanted was not necessarily to keep fasting, but to stay on this healthy path. They had gained traction, they had tasted victory, and they wanted a new life-style. Many wrote that they had been on diet after diet and never had success. Yet on the Daniel Fast they didn't miss food. Cravings disappeared, and they were energized and motivated.

Since then I have hosted many online groups where hundreds of men and women join in a twenty-one-day period of prayer and fasting focusing on health and weight loss. When we focus our attention on God and our desire to please Him, and then also learn how to care better for our bodies, we will almost always achieve success. The rewards go far beyond dropping a few pounds and gaining more energy. We enter into a more personal and intimate relationship with our Lord. We get to know Jesus in a deeper way, and we open our hearts and minds to the Spirit of God as we experience change from the inside out.

What I've discovered is that the best motivation to live a healthier lifestyle doesn't come from a diet book or because we don't like what we see in the mirror. The best incentive is a profound yearning to align our lives with the ways of God and to live according to His desires for us. He wants us to be healthy. He wants us to live vibrant lives. He wants us to be at peace. And He wants us to be positive examples of His children so that others will want what we have: Christ in us.

The apostle Paul writes,

Thanks be to God who always leads us in triumph
in Christ, and through us diffuses the fragrance of

His knowledge in every place. For we are to God the
fragrance of Christ among those who are being saved
and among those who are perishing.

2 CORINTHIANS 2:14-15

As followers of Jesus Christ, we want to be a sweet fragrance for our Lord. We want to bring Him pleasure, and we want to be good examples for the cause of Christ. In our Father's idyllic way, everything that is good for Him is also good for us! So when we devote ourselves to prayer and fasting—even though we may experience some stretching and may need to power through some challenges—the reward on the other side always far outweighs any effort we expend.

ABOUT THE DANIEL FAST

The Daniel Fast is a spiritual experience. If I could shout that statement for all to hear, I would. My heart hurts when I see so many people missing the magnificent benefits of fasting because they focus on the food or turn the fast into a "Christian diet plan." First and foremost, the Daniel Fast is a period of extended prayer that allows us to press into God. We separate ourselves from our typical daily routines and focus more of our time and attention on the Lord and what we need from and through Him. During the fast, we open our hearts to our loving Father. We humble ourselves before Him and learn from Him so we know what to do or how to change.

We'll talk more about this later, but please hear me. While you will almost assuredly drop some unwanted pounds, this is not a diet book. Instead, it's a manual to guide you on a journey toward personal transformation. As part of your spiritual journey, you will learn about yourself, your life in Christ, and how best to treat the physical body that your Creator has entrusted to your care.

God is the designer of fasting, and He designed it with our needs in mind. He knows that at times we need to become more highly focused so we can hear Him better. Fasting is a spiritual discipline for us to use. We don't do it to prove our worth or to show God that we are "good disciples." Jesus is the only One who shows our Father our worth, and that's all been achieved through His blood. As 2 Corinthians 5:21 says, "He made Him who knew no sin to be sin for us, that we might become the righteousness of God in Him."

Neither is the purpose of fasting to change God's mind about something or to make Him love us more. Instead, fasting is a vehicle to change *us*! It's a predetermined period of time in which we consecrate ourselves—set ourselves apart for a spiritual purpose. During this Daniel Fast for Weight Loss, we set ourselves apart from our typical daily life and focus our attention on how God, our Creator, wants us to care for our bodies. Through this process, we experience a transformation that is fueled by desiring to please God and so aligning ourselves with His ways.

The Daniel Fast is a *method* of fasting, rather than a "called fast" that happens at a specific time, such as Passover or Lent. Based on the fasting experiences of the Old Testament prophet Daniel as well as typical Jewish fasting principles, it's a partial fast where some foods are restricted and others are allowed. I encourage you to read *The Daniel Fast: Feed Your Soul, Strengthen Your Spirit, and Renew Your Body*, which was my first book about this method of fasting. In it you will learn much more detailed information about the spiritual discipline of fasting and specifically about the Daniel Fast.

Two passages from the book of Daniel serve as the biblical foundation for the Daniel Fast. First, in Daniel 1 we learn about the young Hebrew man Daniel and his companions, who were in captivity in Babylon during the reign of King Nebuchadnezzar. Babylon's territory was expanding massively, and the kingdom needed more manpower. Nebuchadnezzar took thousands of Hebrews into captivity, including Daniel and his companions. These young men, educated and trained while in Judah, were being groomed for leadership positions.

> *The king [Nebuchadnezzar] instructed Ashpenaz, the master of his eunuchs, to bring some of the children of Israel and some of the king's descendants and some of the nobles, young men in whom there was no blemish, but good-looking, gifted in all wisdom, possessing knowledge and quick to understand, who had ability to serve in the king's palace, and whom they might teach the language and literature of the Chaldeans. And the king appointed for them a daily provision of the king's delicacies and of the wine which he drank, and three years of training for them, so that at the end of that time they might serve before the king.*
>
> DANIEL 1:3-5

Great food. Tasty wine. The very same delicacies that were fit for the king! Sounds tempting, right? But Daniel had something inside of him that was much stronger than his appetite or cravings. He was committed to God, and he wanted to live according to the ways of the Lord.

> *But Daniel purposed in his heart that he would not defile himself with the portion of the king's delicacies, nor with the wine which he drank; therefore he requested of the chief of the eunuchs that he might not defile himself.*
> DANIEL 1:8

Jewish law required meat to be prepared in a very specific manner, which the Babylonians did not follow. In addition, it's likely that King Nebuchadnezzar's food had been offered to the Babylonian gods, and Daniel felt that eating it would make him a participant in idol worship. Even though Daniel was captive in a foreign land, he stood firm in his faith and kept the Hebrew law. He didn't want to defile, or contaminate, his body by eating the food being offered to him.

Here is a point I find precious: Daniel was away from all that was familiar and apart from the community of faith he had known in Israel. Even so, God was still present with him and watching out for him. Daniel 1:9 tells us, "Now God had brought Daniel into the favor and goodwill of the chief of the eunuchs." So when Daniel declined the rich food of the king and asked that he and his friends be given only "pulse" (food grown from seed) to eat and water to drink, the chief of the eunuchs, while reluctant, agreed.

Daniel 1:12 is one of the primary references that establish the guidelines for the Daniel Fast:

Prove thy servants, I beseech thee, ten days; and let them give us pulse to eat, and water to drink. (KJV)

During the fast, we eat only foods grown from seed, including fruits, vegetables, whole grains, legumes, nuts, seeds, healthy oils, spices, and herbs. All food from animals is withheld during the fast, including fish, beef, poultry, dairy products, and eggs. The only beverage on the fast is water. No tea, no coffee, and no juice—just water to comply with this Scripture.

The second reference in the book of Daniel that establishes the guidelines for the Daniel Fast is in Daniel 10. By this time—decades after the events of Daniel 1—Daniel had gone through many trials, but he had also become a leader of great status in Babylon. However, after more than seventy years in captivity, he longed for the day when he could return to Jerusalem and when Israel would once again be a free nation. In much anguish as he hungered for some kind of direction about the future, Daniel turned to extended prayer and fasting. Daniel 10:3 reads,

I ate no pleasant food, no meat or wine came into my mouth, nor did I anoint myself at all, till three whole weeks were fulfilled.

From this Scripture, we glean a few more points about the fast. First, Daniel fasted for twenty-one days. Because of this, most people do the fast and abstain from certain foods for twenty-one consecutive days. Second, Daniel ate no meat, drank no wine, and refrained from eating "pleasant foods."

We use this Scripture (as translated in a variety of Bible versions) to add more restrictions to the Daniel Fast guidelines. These include no sweeteners and no deep-fried foods. Standard Jewish fasting practices, which Daniel most likely followed, also exclude leavening agents. It's possible this is intended by his noting of "no pleasant foods," as many translations specify bread.

From Daniel 1:12 and Daniel 10:3, along with typical Jewish fasting principles, we develop our list of foods consumed while on the Daniel Fast: fruits, vegetables, whole grains, legumes, nuts, seeds, herbs, spices, and healthy oils. The only beverage is water.

The foods not allowed on the Daniel Fast are any that are produced from animals or that include leavening agents, solid fats, sweeteners (either natural or artificial), chemicals, food additives, preservatives, or processed ingredients. Also, no deep-fried foods.

A more extensive list of allowed foods is included in the recipe section of this book, along with some tips for preparing meals. But please, don't rush off there.

DON'T SETTLE FOR LESS AND MISS THE BEST

In our fast and furious culture of instant diet solutions for painless weight loss, so often we rush off to the quick and easy solution. Our society's messages train us to skip ahead. Use the CliffsNotes. Take the easy way so you'll have the instant results you are looking for. Sometimes those quick and easy options are helpful, like when you need to clean a stain in your carpet or find the best route to a location you've never visited before. But here, when it comes to discovering some of the mysteries of our faith, you don't want the quick and easy way. You don't want to skip ahead to the recipes and menus and miss the life-changing truths that your Lord wants you to understand. Don't settle for less (the quick and easy) and miss the best (the lasting and true).

Jesus calls us to a new way of life. He says, "The time is fulfilled, and the kingdom of God is at hand. Repent, and believe in the gospel" (Mark 1:15). The word *repent* in the Greek is *metanoeo*, which means "change, transfigure, transform, or reconsider." Our Lord is calling us to a new way of being that He has made possible by coming into the world, redeeming us, and restoring us to the Father. He tells us to "believe in the gospel." We need to learn about this new way of living that He's made possible and then entrench these new truths into every part of who we are. We want to make His ways our ways so we can live this new life in Christ!

In John 14:21 Jesus says, "He who has My commandments and keeps them, it is he who loves Me. And he who loves Me will be loved by My Father, and I will love him and manifest Myself to him." *Manifest* means to show up or to declare wisdom through words. Can you grasp this amazing privilege we have at hand? The One who upholds "all things by the word of His power" (Hebrews 1:3) makes Himself available to you and me and anyone who will keep His commandments. Jesus shows Himself to us, and we express our love to Him by doing what He says to do. We learn His teachings from the Scriptures and then we make the necessary changes in our lives so we are aligned with Him. Our way of living becomes consistent with the heart of our Savior.

This is the Christian life. This is Kingdom of God living. This is the life of a thankful and humble servant like Paul described to the Galatians: "I have been crucified with Christ and I no longer live, but Christ lives in me. The life I now live in the body, I live by faith in the Son of God, who loved me and gave himself for me" (2:20, NIV).

Our beloved epistle writer Paul shares how to live this way:

> *I beseech you therefore, brethren, by the mercies of God,*
> *that you present your bodies a living sacrifice, holy,*
> *acceptable to God, which is your reasonable service. And*
> *do not be conformed to this world, but be transformed*
> *by the renewing of your mind, that you may prove what*
> *is that good and acceptable and perfect will of God.*
> ROMANS 12:1-2

The Daniel Fast serves as a powerful tool that can help you focus on God and His Word, renew your mind, and experience the changes you want to see in yourself. These changes will bring you closer to God and will help you crucify your flesh—that part of you that is not aligned with God. The Bible says:

> *What the law could not do in that it was weak through*
> *the flesh, God did by sending His own Son in the*

*likeness of sinful flesh, on account of sin: He condemned
sin in the flesh, that the righteous requirement of the
law might be fulfilled in us who do not walk according
to the flesh but according to the Spirit. For those who
live according to the flesh set their minds on the things
of the flesh, but those who live according to the Spirit,
the things of the Spirit.*

ROMANS 8:3-5

One of the most valuable lessons we can learn on the
Daniel Fast is how to suppress the influence of our flesh,
or human nature, through submission and obedience. By
setting our minds on the things of the Spirit, we allow the
Spirit of God living in us to have more power in our lives.
Our ultimate goal is to be Spirit-led rather than led by our
flesh.

I am filled with joy when I hear from people who have
been profoundly touched by God during their fast as they
experienced this transformation. I often find myself in tears
as I read messages from believers who have developed a
deeper relationship with Jesus during their fast, who have
been reconciled with a loved one, or who have experienced
breakthroughs in financial matters. Others have discovered
self-control and a desire to develop a healthy lifestyle as they
submit all of who they are to God and adopt new habits
that become their way of living. Oh, my heart bursts with
joy and thanksgiving when I hear the testimonies of God
working in the lives of His people to bring blessing, hope,
and health!

Unfortunately, there is another side of this coin. I also read messages from people who become so focused on the "letter of the law"—what food items are allowed or not allowed on the fast—that they miss the deep truths available for them. Over the last couple of years I've seen the promotion of "delectable Daniel Fast meals," "mouth-watering Daniel Fast recipes," and "tempting Daniel Fast dessert recipes that will satisfy your sweet tooth." Can you see what these are all doing? They are serving the flesh, and that is contrary to what our Christian life is about. God has created the spiritual discipline of fasting so His people can draw closer to Him and receive blessings and answers to prayer. To turn that into a way to pamper your taste buds while still maintaining the rules of the fast completely cancels the purpose of fasting.

The Daniel Fast is indeed a very healthy way to eat. But fasting is not about figuring out ways to satisfy our bodies while still upholding the guidelines of the fast. It's about submitting ourselves to God so that He can fill us! My hope is that you will not go for the easy way of the flesh and miss out on the best that God has for you.

Does that mean you will consume only tasteless, boring foods on the fast? Are you wrong if you enjoy the meals you prepare? No. It's okay to make Daniel Fast–compliant menus that will nourish your body and be pleasant to your palate. The key is to keep the food in its appropriate place—and that's off the pedestal that so many of us have it on. You will find this balanced approach throughout this book, and it's a key to developing your own lifestyle of health.

The Daniel Fast is a vehicle that allows you to receive the amazing truths that the Lord eagerly wants to give you as you draw near to Him. During your Daniel Fast, you will learn how to put your sinful nature in its humble position and become stronger in your spirit as you walk according to the Spirit of God. I'll share more about this very essential issue in chapter 6. My hope for right now is that as you open your mind and heart to this fasting experience, you will start out on the right foot! Don't set yourself up for a mediocre or disappointing fasting experience. Instead, choose the path that leads to spiritual growth, renewal, and transformation as you focus on what God wants for your health—a transformation that can last for your whole life and not just for twenty-one days.

During your Daniel Fast you'll find yourself turning away from food and turning toward God. All along you'll eat healthy foods for an extended period of time—in fact, you'll eat the very foods your Creator designed to nourish the body He designed. You'll get off the sugar roller coaster and soon find a new level of energy.

As you partner with your loving Father, you'll begin to change from the inside out as you embrace your identity as a valuable child of the Most High God. You will experience freedom from the bondages of food, overeating, cravings, and fatigue that may have become your normal life. You will soon have a new normal, but this one will be based on living a faith-driven life for health and well-being.

BEFORE YOU BEGIN

The Daniel Fast includes a very healthy eating plan. However, please allow the Great Physician to work hand in hand with your earthly physician. Any time you enter into a significant change to your diet and exercise routines, it's a good idea to check with your health professional for his or her input.

Fasting should never harm the body. If you have special dietary needs—if you are pregnant or nursing, if you have a chronic illness such as cancer or diabetes, if you are a young person who is still growing or an athlete who expends more than typical amounts of energy on a regular basis—contact your health professional and modify the Daniel Fast eating plan in a way that is appropriate to meet your health needs.

HOW TO USE THIS BOOK

This book will give you practical help as you prepare for the Daniel Fast, go through it, and transition out of it. I recommend that you read at least through chapter 2 before you begin your fast, as it will walk you through the specifics of planning menus, buying food, and preparing yourself for the fasting experience.

The remainder of the book can be read either before you begin the fast or as you are doing it. Chapters 3 and 4 lay the scriptural foundation for how we should view our bodies, chapter 5 discusses the specific health benefits of the fast, and chapter 6 deals with physical and spiritual responses to food cravings and broader temptations. Chapters 7 through 9 will guide you as you complete the fast and think about what changes you want to make as you transition into a healthier lifestyle both physically and spiritually.

You'll also find other significant helps later in the book. I've included a number of recipes for breakfasts, lunches, dinners, and snacks that will give you ideas of how to cook healthy, satisfying foods within the Daniel Fast guidelines. (Recipes that are particularly low in calories are marked with a special icon.) You will also find a twenty-one-day devotional that will offer spiritual support as you go through the fast. If you need more help, visit my blog at danielfast.wordpress.com. You'll find plenty of articles, answers to common questions, and practical tips to get you through the fast successfully.

It's been my privilege to share in the fasting journeys of thousands of people over the past several years. My prayer is that as you begin the Daniel Fast seeking weight loss and improved health, you will be blessed in spirit, soul, and body.

WEIGHT LOSS SUCCESS TIP

Before you eat something—especially if you feel you are caving to temptations—pause for a few minutes. Don't take a bite, but instead candidly talk to the Lord. Humble yourself before Him and renew your commitment to follow His good ways for your life. You will be surprised how this simple step will alleviate almost all those times when you consume foods you really don't want to eat.

CHAPTER 2

Get Ready

*Preparing for the Fast
Mentally, Spiritually, and Physically*

CAN YOU REMEMBER A TIME when you went on a vacation or to an event, and your experience was much grander than you had ever envisioned? You were surprised by the joy you felt and the fun you had—and it was even better because it was all unexpected.

I was able to give an unexpected experience to my sister Nancy and her husband, Ron, a few years ago. Nancy had recently recovered from breast cancer, which was complicated by some other medical issues. She was healthy again but still had not regained her total strength.

She told me about an upcoming vacation to Puerto Vallarta that she and Ron had planned. The small, quaint resort where they would stay is one where I stay for my annual writing retreat. I've been going there for decades and know the place inside and out. Many of the staff members have become dear friends, including Eduardo, the front desk manager, and Charo in guest services.

When I was sure of my sister's travel dates, I started to make plans. I knew that every Monday afternoon at 5:00, the resort hosts a welcome party for the guests. I knew that Nancy and Ron would attend, so I surreptitiously planned with Eduardo and Charo to create a romantic four-course candlelit dinner on the beach for my sister and her husband.

After the welcome party was underway, Charo told Nancy and Ron that she had a surprise for them. She took them both by the hand and led them down to the shore to reveal their private beach dinner. The resort staff had constructed a lovely gauze canopy that blew gently in the sea breeze. They had arranged a table for two, set with fine china and glassware, and then added a beautiful tropical flower arrangement for a centerpiece. The hotel chef had planned a gourmet menu, and a guitarist was on hand to serenade the couple during their romantic dining experience. Nancy and Ron took their seats, the servers delivered their first course, and the guitar player strummed his instrument. It was an enchanting evening on the beach.

Nancy and Ron thought they were only going to a welcome party hosted by the resort. They had no idea that a surprise awaited them—one that was planned especially for them and would deliver so much joy, delight, and pleasure. All they needed to do was to walk into the experience.

The same is true for you, particularly if this is your first time using the Daniel Fast. You may know some of the details of the fast and the framework of the discipline, but you don't know what your loving Father already has planned for you as you open your heart and submit yourself to Him. I encourage you to get ready for what is to come. Do your part by being prepared spiritually, mentally, and physically, even though you don't yet know the whole picture of what's ahead.

I am so glad Nancy and Ron didn't skip the welcome party or make plans to be somewhere else at the very time their surprise was delivered to them. They needed to be in the right place at the right time. And I say the same for you. Be ready for your fast so your Lord can give you the blessings and gifts He has already prepared for you.

SET YOURSELF UP FOR SUCCESS

More than you know awaits you, and you'll discover it during your Daniel Fast. Your blessings will be both physical and spiritual. As you study and meditate on His Word, the Holy Spirit will reveal truth to your spirit and increase your understanding. Your spiritual ears will be quickened during your quiet time with Him as you become more intent on hearing that still, small voice that speaks inside of you. The Lord will bare insights for you as you seek His wisdom about your life and your well-being.

Because one purpose for your Daniel Fast is to gain greater health and drop unwanted pounds, you'll also increase in knowledge about healthy eating principles you can live by and carry into your future. As you follow the Daniel Fast and experience it with your spirit, soul, and body, you'll begin a transformation. Day by day and step by step you'll gain traction and strength.

One way of looking at your Daniel Fast for Weight Loss is as a spiritual journey. It's similar to long-distance walking in that you start at one place (your current physical state) and continue to move toward where you want to go (a lifestyle of health and well-being). Your journey can transform your life as you forge on and move forward one step at a time.

In 2011, I embarked on a long-distance walking journey— called *el Camino de Santiago*—that changed my life forever. It's a five-hundred-mile pilgrimage that starts in France, continues across northern Spain, and finishes in Santiago, which is near the western coast of the country. I knew the basics of what I would do during the journey. I knew that each day I would walk between twelve and fifteen miles. I would eat at restaurants and small cafes along the way, and I would sleep in *refugios*, which are like hostels that are reserved only for those walking the Camino.

I was prepared with the appropriate equipment, including a backpack, walking shoes, and walking poles. I had the right water bottles, clothes, and toiletries. I had also prepared my body by embarking on many long-distance training walks. In fact, I had studied the Camino ever since I added it to my "lifetime experience" list more than twelve years earlier. I knew all about the Camino de Santiago, but now I was actually entering into the experience.

The first few days were grueling as my body got used to using muscles that weren't as strong as they needed to be. While I had trained for long-distance walking, I wasn't prepared for the steep climb from Saint-Jean-Pied-de-Port in France, up the Pyrenees Mountains into Spain, and then on to Roncesvalles, which at its highest point is more than 4,100 feet—all in two days.

However, even more unexpected were the amazing gifts and treasures I received over my thirty-six consecutive days of walking. None of these priceless rewards were physical items. Instead, they were new cherished friendships with others walking the Camino. They were amazing insights about me and my relationship with my Lord, discovered as I spent many hours walking in silence to the world, yet in deep conversation with Him. They were breathtaking views as my eyes absorbed God's artistry in the changing landscapes of mountains, forests, and valleys. I received precious gifts of love and encouragement—some in smiles and others in offerings of food or water—from men, women, and children who lived on the Camino pathway. Most precious were the inward gifts of personal satisfaction and gratitude to God for a fulfilled goal and hope.

Valuable lessons. Priceless gifts. Splendid memories. And they all came through the action of walking the Camino de Santiago.

You are about to begin a journey of a different type, but you also will receive many unforeseen treasures. You want to be ready. You want to be prepared. You want to have an open heart to absorb all that the Lord wants to give you as you take your first step toward revelation, transformation, and renewal.

PREPARE YOUR HEART

Proverbs 4:23 says, "Guard your heart above all else, for it determines the course of your life" (NLT). This is a truth we can use in everything we do and say! Your attitude and your mind-set can determine the course of your fasting experience. Taking the time to decide intentionally how you will approach this discipline will have a major effect on the benefits you will receive from your time of extended prayer and fasting.

So many people jump into the fast without preparing their hearts, or they engage only half-heartedly. It reminds me of a woman I know through a business association. She is smart and knows so much about publishing information over the Internet. Over the last five years she has invested tens of thousands of dollars and hundreds of hours to learn the latest techniques and the powerful systems now available. She attends all our association meetings, and she can hold her own in a conversation about websites. But the truth is, she has remained on the sidelines. She's never really entered the game as a player. She has studied. She has learned. She has talked. But she has never published a website or used her knowledge to make a difference in the lives of those she can serve.

I often see the same type of behavior with people who fast. They read about fasting, and they may even use the Daniel Fast as their method and change what they eat. However, they stay only on the surface, rather than submitting themselves more fully to the Lord and going deep with Him as they fast.

Another mistake I see people make is that they wait for God to do something. Rather than developing a purpose for their fast and asking God to work in their hearts and circumstances, they stay in a passive position, just waiting to see what God will do in their lives.

A third mistake is focusing on the negatives instead of

the positives. I hear from many people who whine about the foods they will miss or murmur about the hardship the fast will be on their lives. When their thoughts are centered on what they're going to give up during the fast instead of what they might gain, they miss the point.

I encourage a different approach to your fast. Even now as you begin to prepare your mind and heart for the twenty-one-day experience, decide that you will join in with all your might. Decide to fully embrace the experience and draw near to your loving Father so He can indeed draw near to you. It's like getting onto a tennis court or a football field. If you play in a passive, mediocre way, you might not get very tired. But if you really want to improve, you'll give it all you have and do your best. That's the approach you need when you fast if you want this powerful spiritual discipline to be effective in your life.

When you fast, you need to enter into the experience. I like to think of it as crossing a threshold and being in a different realm for an extended period of time. It's like going on a personal spiritual retreat, but you don't have to leave your home, take a leave from work, or delay fulfilling your responsibilities. In fact, one of the main benefits of the Daniel Fast is that you can be "in the experience" while still carrying on your duties and daily activities. It's a shadow of how we are as believers. Jesus pronounces in John 17:14-15 that His followers are in the world but not of it, and during your Daniel Fast you can be more conscious of this existence. While you "live in" the spiritual realm of fasting, you still continue in your everyday life.

When you enter into your fast, you cross the threshold. Even in the first days, you may sense the Spirit of God placing a covering on you. It's like a protective cocoon or a shielding robe, and it comes as you draw nearer to God and focus more of your time and attention on Him.

SET ASIDE THE TIME

One of the biggest practical considerations when getting ready for a fast is deciding when your fast will start and when it will end. You may be following the fast with others in your church or study group. If so, the dates are already set. But if you are planning the fast on your own, take a look at your calendar and find a time that is free of big events, extended travel, or other activities that could interfere with your fast. Try to imagine yourself in the fasting experience, including setting aside additional time for prayer, study, meditation, and being with your Lord.

You'll also want to anticipate added time for planning and preparing meals. I'll share some proven success tips in the recipe section for organizing meal plans and making this process easier. If you are not accustomed to preparing most of your meals from scratch in your own kitchen, you'll want to step back and see how you can arrange your weekly and daily activities so you'll have the time.

If the thought of preparing your own meals sends a shiver up your spine, please relax. The meals I suggest are simple to prepare, plus I also give ideas for creating multiple meals in one cooking session so you cook once, but eat several times. These are good plans to use not only during your fast, but all the time as you turn away from prepared meals that are higher in calories and often lower in nutrition.

You want to be at the top of your game during your fast. Plan to get adequate sleep and rest so you can enter into the peace that Jesus offers you. These days should reflect the life our Savior provides when we live according to His ways and accept His invitation:

> *Come to Me, all you who labor and are heavy laden, and I will give you rest. Take My yoke upon you and learn from Me, for I am gentle and lowly in heart, and you will find rest for your souls. For My yoke is easy and My burden is light.*
> MATTHEW 11:28-30

Holy Days

The word *holy* means "separated for the purposes of God." Your period of extended prayer and fasting will consist of holy days—days separated for a spiritual purpose.

Fasting isn't a new layer of activity to add to already busy days. Just as the early church created seasons for Christian observance, your fast is your special time. It's a set-aside time of consecration.

Think of your twenty-one holy days as ones where you control the use of your time. Make intentional choices about what you will and won't do rather than allowing your busy schedule or the demands on your life to control you. During your time of consecration, take charge of your days. As Jesus teaches us, "Seek first the kingdom of God and His righteousness, and all these things shall be added to you" (Matthew 6:33). Begin with God's Kingdom and His way of doing things as you start each day, and move from this starting point—not just during your fast but in all your life.

PREPARE YOUR BODY

The Daniel Fast includes a very healthy eating plan. You will be well-nourished as you give your body the foods it wants to function as it was designed. However, if you typically consume caffeine or a lot of sugary foods, you will want to prepare your body so you will be ready on the first day of your fast.

Listen up, users of coffee, tea, and other caffeinated beverages and foods: You want to avoid caffeine withdrawal, as it can be debilitating. A 2004 report from Johns Hopkins Medicine states: "In general, the more caffeine consumed, the more severe withdrawal symptoms are likely to be, but as little as one standard cup of coffee a day can produce caffeine addiction, according to a Johns Hopkins study that reviewed over 170 years of caffeine withdrawal research."[1]

In the report, Roland Griffiths, PhD, professor of psychiatry and neuroscience at Johns Hopkins, says, "The latest research demonstrates, however, that when people don't get their usual dose [of caffeine] they can suffer a range of withdrawal symptoms, including headache, fatigue, [and] difficulty concentrating. They may even feel like they have the flu with nausea and muscle pain."[2]

If you are a user of caffeine, plan to taper off the drug (yes, it is considered a drug) seven to ten days before you begin your fast. Begin by increasing the amount of water you drink and by substituting your normal caffeinated beverages with half-caf for two to five days. (That's half regular coffee or tea with half decaffeinated coffee or tea.) Follow this with two to three days of a 25-75 blend, or 25 percent regular coffee or tea with 75 percent decaffeinated coffee or tea. Finally, for one to two days, drink only decaf. Then on the first day of your fast you should be ready to comply with the Daniel Fast guidelines and drink only water for your beverage.

The Daniel Fast is also high in fiber. Fiber is the part of fruits and vegetables that cannot be digested; however, it's of vital importance to digestion. Fiber helps the body move food through the digestive tract, and acts like a sponge to soak up extra cholesterol that would otherwise return to the bloodstream. This is the primary reason that some on the Daniel Fast report lowering their LDL cholesterol. With the increase of fiber, the body can function as God intended it, using the foods He created for us. Fiber also contributes to disease protection.

If you are not accustomed to eating a lot of fiber-rich foods, you may want to begin introducing more of them into your meals before the fast begins so your digestive system can be trained to manage the elements. Add fiber gradually over a few weeks to avoid abdominal discomfort caused by the bacteria in your digestive system. Drinking plenty of water aids the passage of fiber and can reduce discomfort.

Plan Your Menus and Your Mealtimes

You will likely prepare most of your Daniel Fast meals and snacks at home since so few of the prepared offerings from restaurants, drive-throughs, and supermarket shelves comply with the fasting guidelines. This may be a great time to develop new healthy habits as you become more conscious about the foods you consume and invest time and energy into creating meals that serve your body rather than bring it harm or cause weight gain.

If you commonly don't prepare many of your own meals, don't let this become a burden. Instead, plan to use this time as part of your fasting experience. Even though cooking isn't a passion for me, I do find myself preparing my Daniel Fast meals with a dominance of joy, enthusiasm, and thanksgiving. I usually prepare several meals at one time so I can multiply the results of each minute in the kitchen. During my cooking time, I often crank up the volume on praise music or listen to an audio teaching by one of my favorite pastors, authors, or Bible teachers. Knowing I am working to bring good to my body, that I am accomplishing a lot of work in a short period of time, and that I am growing spiritually while doing it all makes cooking a pleasant experience. Plus, the time passes so quickly that before I know it I have four or five meals prepared (some stored in the freezer) and I'm full of joy and gratitude.

Having appropriate food on hand during your Daniel Fast also contributes to your success. So as you prepare to begin, make sure you have snacks in your cupboard or fridge that are ready when you want them. I've included many options in the recipe section of this book.

You'll also want to have what I call "fast food" for your Daniel Fast. These are meals that can be prepared in less time than it takes to have a pizza delivered to your door. You'll want to have the recipes on hand and the ingredients available. You can also have frozen meals ready to defrost and prepare in minutes. One of my standards is a vegetarian chili that I've made for decades, even before I used the Daniel Fast. I make the chili year-round in large batches so I have some for lunches and dinner, plus extra for the freezer. I just defrost the frozen chili and serve it with a green salad from the washed and cut vegetables I keep in the fridge. Within fifteen to twenty minutes I am sitting down to a satisfying, nutritious, and Daniel Fast–compliant meal.

You'll want to plan your own quick meals. It's kind of like investing in insurance. Rather than breaking the fast because you're too tired or too rushed to cook, you can plan ahead, prepare your "fast food," and remain on the fast.

Stocking the Pantry

Even before you begin your fast, you can start stocking up for it. You might even be able to take advantage of grocery-store bargains. Here are just a few of the items I keep on hand in my cupboards:

- all-natural peanut butter
- boxed unsweetened soy milk
- boxed vegetable broth
- brown rice
- canned "lite" fruit
- canned beans

- canned chili peppers
- canned tomatoes
- canned tomato sauce
- dried fruit
- garlic
- muesli whole grain cereal
- nuts
- olive oil
- onions
- quinoa
- rice cakes
- tahini (to make hummus)
- tamari sauce
- seasonings
- whole grain pasta

I also stock my refrigerator and freezer with some staples:

- carrots
- celery
- cucumbers
- green onions
- green peppers
- frozen corn
- frozen peas
- lemons
- mixed lettuce
- radishes
- red peppers

These ingredients can be the makings for quick break-fasts, lunches, dinners, and snacks. And since I have fast and easy recipes at my fingertips—including herbed red sauce with pasta, vegetarian chili, hot muesli with soy milk, rice cakes with peanut butter and raisins, or black bean hummus with veggies—I am always prepared and able to stay within the fasting guidelines, no matter what comes up.

Just as the Girl and Boy Scouts recommend, you want to "be prepared."

- Prepare your mind and heart
- Prepare your time
- Prepare your body
- Prepare your food supplies
- Prepare for your meals

In the next two chapters we'll take a deeper look at biblical truths about our bodies. We'll discover how to push aside the lies we often believe and cling to the amazing truth that our bodies are dwelling places of God.

Set yourself up for success by preparing yourself for what can be a powerful transformative experience for your life and your health. Ready? Let's go!

WEIGHT LOSS SUCCESS TIP

Take a time-out from reading for a few minutes and think about your physical body. Consider all the things it does, including walking, lifting, working, and playing. Consider its inner workings: the blood that flows through your veins, your digestive system, and your joints and muscles. Thank God for creating you and for masterfully designing and constructing your body. Form a habit of expressing gratitude for it throughout the day. You will soon see how these simple steps will foster in you a desire to care for yourself.

CHAPTER 3

A Dwelling Place for God

What the Bible Tells Us about Our Bodies

You ARE READING what may be the most important chapter of this book. My hope is that as you read these words, you will begin to understand a powerful truth about who you are as a born-again follower of Jesus Christ. Through this knowledge, I pray that you will more fully appreciate your identity and the way you can live in Christ.

I want to guide you through a brief study of Old and New Testament truths about God, His love for people, His great desire to be among us, and what that means for you today as you learn about your body, your health, and how to live each day according to God's truth about you.

The Bible teaches us the value God places on knowledge and understanding:

> *My son, if you receive my words,*
> *And treasure my commands within you,*

So that you incline your ear to wisdom,
And apply your heart to understanding;
Yes, if you cry out for discernment,
And lift up your voice for understanding,
If you seek her as silver,
And search for her as for hidden treasures;
Then you will understand the fear of the LORD,
And find the knowledge of God.
For the LORD *gives wisdom;*
From His mouth come knowledge and understanding.

PROVERBS 2:1-6

Knowledge and understanding from God are the precursors to His wisdom. We gain knowledge through study, and then we reap wisdom by opening our hearts and minds to the truths we've learned through God's precepts. Understanding soaks into our souls and causes us to think through the prism of what we have learned. Understanding forms our beliefs, and out of those beliefs come our behaviors. This is why God's instruction to us is this: "Wisdom is the principal thing; therefore get wisdom. And in all your getting, get understanding" (Proverbs 4:7).

What we believe to be true informs how we live. That's why it's so important that we understand how God views our bodies, because if we believe that they are good and valuable in His eyes, we will learn to treat them that way. Jesus says, "Take my yoke upon you and learn from Me, for I am gentle and lowly in heart, and you will find rest for your souls" (Matthew 11:29). When we learn from the Master, we receive the understanding we need so we can live the life He promises. By digging into God's truth found in His Word, then meditating on it so we receive revelation and understanding, we are able to find the rest our souls long for. That is the secure life. The Kingdom life.

OUR CONNECTION WITH GOD

In this chapter, I want to help you gain understanding about your body. I'm not talking about anatomy or science. Rather, I want you to know the truth about the spiritual transformation your body underwent when you made Jesus the Lord of your life.

Here is what God's precious Word says about your body: "Do you not know that you are the temple of God and that the Spirit of God dwells in you?" (1 Corinthians 3:16). It's easy to read those words and then move on, but I encourage you to pause. Read the words again and think about the truth God reveals to you through them.

You—the very body that bears the eyes you are using to read these words; the body that supports the fingers you're using to turn the pages; the physical body that houses your spirit and your soul—also house the Spirit of God.

His Spirit is always with you. Deuteronomy 31:6 says, "Be strong and of good courage, do not fear nor be afraid of them; for the LORD your God, He is the One who goes with you. He will not leave you nor forsake you." When God initially made that promise, it was to Joshua, who was to lead His chosen people from the wilderness into the Promised Land. But this truth has remained the same throughout all time: God loves

His people so much that He wants to be with them. That has been His desire from the first days of creation when He said, "Let Us make man in Our image" (Genesis 1:26). The Lord and His created beings shared an intimate relationship. God cared for His people, and He created a perfect home for Adam and Eve where they could be with Him, to talk and walk together in the cool of the day (see Genesis 2:8; 3:8).

But then sin broke the intimate connection God shared with Adam and Eve. Their Creator had warned them that they would die if they disobeyed: "The LORD God commanded the man, saying, 'Of every tree of the garden you may freely eat; but of the tree of the knowledge of good and evil you shall not eat, for in the day that you eat of it you shall surely die'" (Genesis 2:16-17). When they listened to Satan instead of God, they ate fruit from the forbidden tree. Adam and Eve didn't experience physical death at that moment, but the ceaseless and intimate spiritual connection they had with the Spirit of God died immediately—for them and for all humans after them.

Even after that broken relationship, God continued to work with His created people to renew the deep, innermost connection they had lost. He desired to live among those He had chosen. When God gave Moses the Law at Sinai, God instructed him to make a tabernacle for a meeting place where God might dwell with His people. He told Moses, "Let them make Me a sanctuary, that I may dwell among them. According to all that I show you, that is, the pattern of the tabernacle and the pattern of all its furnishings, just so you shall make it" (Exodus 25:8-9).

The Tabernacle of Meeting, or the Tabernacle in the Wilderness, was first constructed in approximately 1250 BC. The word *tabernacle* means "dwelling place," and this structure would be the dwelling place of God in the midst of His chosen people. The Tabernacle in the Wilderness was a holy place set apart for the purposes of God, including prayer, worship, sacrifices, and meeting with Him. God's instructions for how to construct this portable dwelling place were intricately detailed, with specific functions for each part. He also stipulated that the best of materials should be used. Not only were they sturdy enough to hold up to the elements, but they were beautiful to the eye. Beauty is appropriate for the home of God.

God also assigned caretakers for His Tabernacle—His home. He commanded Aaron, Moses' older brother and God's high priest among men, to be the caretaker of the Tabernacle along with his sons and descendants, as we see in these passages from Exodus.

> *In the tabernacle of meeting, outside the veil which is before the Testimony, Aaron and his sons shall tend [the lamp] from evening until morning before the LORD. It shall be a statute forever to their generations on behalf of the children of Israel.*
>
> EXODUS 27:21

> *I will consecrate the tabernacle of meeting and the altar. I will also consecrate both Aaron and his sons to minister to Me as priests.*
>
> EXODUS 29:44

The Tabernacle, surrounded by a fenced outer court, was comprised of two compartments, which were separated by a thick, heavy curtain called a veil. The inner compartment, behind the veil, was called the Most Holy Place and served as the dwelling place of God. In this space was the Ark of the Covenant, which held the two tablets of the Law that were written by the finger of God and given to Moses on Mount Sinai, a jar of manna, and Aaron's rod, which budded and bore fruit (see Exodus 31:18; Hebrews 9:3-4).

Atop the Ark were two golden cherubim with outstretched wings. Between them was the mercy seat, and it was above this that the presence of God lived. God told Moses:

> *There I will meet with you, and I will speak with you from above the mercy seat, from between the two cherubim which are on the ark of the Testimony, about everything which I will give you in commandment to the children of Israel.*
> EXODUS 25:22

> *You shall hang the veil from the clasps. Then you shall bring the ark of the Testimony in there, behind the veil. The veil shall be a divider for you between the holy place and the Most Holy.*
> EXODUS 26:33

Only the high priest was allowed to enter behind the veil, and even then just once every year on the Day of Atonement, or Yom Kippur, which is the holiest day of the year for the

Jewish people. In Leviticus 16:2, the Lord instructed Moses, "Tell Aaron your brother not to come at just any time into the Holy Place inside the veil, before the mercy seat which is on the ark, lest he die; for I will appear in the cloud above the mercy seat."

God took special care to design and plan His dwelling place. He selected those who would take care of His residence and gave them clear, detailed instructions to follow as they offered sacrifices for the people. Aaron was the high priest to God and the caretaker of the very place God chose to live.

THE TEMPLE IN JERUSALEM

Later, the portable Tabernacle in the Wilderness was replaced with a permanent dwelling for God. It was the Temple in Jerusalem, designed by David and constructed under the authority of his son Solomon in about 968 BC. The priests followed the same instructions that had been established by God, and His holy presence was again in the midst of His chosen people. In 1 Kings 8 we read about God's glory in the Temple:

> It came to pass, when the priests came out of the holy place, that the cloud filled the house of the LORD, so that the priests could not continue ministering because of the cloud; for the glory of the LORD filled the house of the LORD.
> I KINGS 8:10-11

Solomon's Temple remained the center of worship and sacrifice for God's chosen people until King Nebuchadnezzar of Babylon destroyed it in 586 BC. This was the same time that Daniel was taken captive during the Babylonian exile.

It wasn't until 515 BC that another Temple was constructed in Jerusalem under the leadership of Zerubbabel, who led the first wave of captives from Babylon back to their home in Judah. This Temple was dismantled nearly five hundred years later when Jerusalem was under Roman rule, and it was replaced in AD 19 by what was called Herod's Temple. This is the Temple that we read about during Jesus' time on earth.

THE SEPARATION IS OVER

When Jesus came to earth, everything changed for the future of humankind. People had been separated from God because of the sin that entered the world in the Garden of Eden through Adam and Eve's dreadful choice. But God longed for reconciliation, and on that first Christmas morning more than two thousand years ago, the settlement began. It was announced to the shepherds watching over their sheep by night: "Suddenly there was with the angel a multitude of the heavenly host praising God and saying: 'Glory to God in the highest, and on earth peace, goodwill toward men!'" (Luke 2:13-14). A Savior had been born, and reconciliation with God was on its way.

During Jesus' ministry on earth, He continually preached that everything was now different for anyone who believed. We read in Matthew 4:17, "From that time Jesus began to preach and to say, 'Repent, for the kingdom of heaven is at hand.'" *At hand* means it's right here for you to receive.

When we change our way of thinking (repent), we find that an entirely new way of living is available.

Jesus told many parables about the value of God's Kingdom. In Matthew 13:45-46 we read His words: "The kingdom of heaven is like a merchant seeking beautiful pearls, who, when he had found one pearl of great price, went and sold all that he had and bought it." You, dear one, are a pearl of great price in the mind of your Creator. He loves you so much that He gave dearly to be rejoined with you. One of the most famous verses in the Bible states this beautifully: "For God so loved the world that He gave His only begotten Son, that whoever believes in Him should not perish but have everlasting life" (John 3:16).

God gave His only Son out of love for us and His unending desire to be reconciled to us. He wanted to end the separation caused by sin. It was at the Cross that the dissolution of another separation took place: the one represented by the heavy veil that kept people from God's presence in the Most Holy Place—where only the high priest was allowed to enter one time a year on the Day of Atonement. Matthew 27 tells the story vividly:

> *Jesus cried out again with a loud voice, and yielded up His spirit.*
> *Then, behold, the veil of the temple was torn in two from top to bottom; and the earth quaked, and the rocks were split, and the graves were opened; and many bodies of the saints who had fallen asleep were raised.*
> MATTHEW 27:50-52

When Jesus sacrificed Himself on the cross, God changed His dwelling place among people. He is no longer confined only to the Temple; instead, He now offers to take up residence in our hearts. The most dramatic example of this came on the Day of Pentecost, when the Holy Spirit filled all the believers and enabled them to preach boldly to people of all nations (see Acts 2). One of these believers, Stephen, later preached to the Pharisees about God's true dwelling place:

> *Solomon built Him a house.*
> *However, the Most High does not dwell in temples made with hands, as the prophet says:*
>
> > *"Heaven is My throne,*
> > *And earth is My footstool.*
> > *What house will you build for Me? says the LORD,*
> > *Or what is the place of My rest?"*
>
> ACTS 7:47-49

God no longer dwells in human-made temples, but each of us can invite Him into our hearts. Revelation 3:20 records Jesus' words: "Behold, I stand at the door and knock. If anyone hears My voice and opens the door, I will come in to him and dine with him, and he with Me."

Through this act of inviting Jesus into our hearts, we become the home of God—the very place where He lives with us. We now are the temple, made not by human hands but by the hand of God. As we saw already in the apostle Paul's first letter to the Corinthians,

Do you not know that you are the temple of God and
that the Spirit of God dwells in you? If anyone defiles
the temple of God, God will destroy him. For the temple
of God is holy, which temple you are.

1 CORINTHIANS 3:16-17

I hope you are allowing these truths to seep into your understanding. These are not just opinions; this is the truth of God communicated to us through His Word. If you are a believer in Christ, God is in you. *You* are His dwelling place.

When you invite the Lord into your life, your spirit is born again and reconciled with the Spirit of God. You can have an intimate connection with Him, just as Adam and Eve did before sin entered the world. The big difference for us is that our soul—the "natural man" part of us—has already been trained by the world's way of doing things. Our lives as followers of Jesus involve aligning any part of that worldly thinking with the truth that comes only from the Son of God. Jesus said,

I am the way, the truth, and the life. No one comes
to the Father except through Me. . . . If anyone loves
Me, he will keep My word; and My Father will
love him, and We will come to him and make Our
home with him.

JOHN 14:6, 23

Our spirit is rejoined with God's Holy Spirit, and we are called to live according to the teachings of Jesus, who speaks only what His Father has told Him. In John 12:49 Jesus says, "For I have not spoken on My own authority; but the Father who sent Me gave Me a command, what I should say and what I should speak." We can have confidence in His words.

Our role, as faithful followers and partakers of the heavenly Kingdom that He made possible, is to set ourselves apart for God's purposes by learning His ways. We are called to sanctify ourselves for Him. Paul writes in 1 Thessalonians 5:23, "Now may the God of peace Himself sanctify you completely; and may your whole spirit, soul, and body be preserved blameless at the coming of our Lord Jesus Christ."

That change—becoming sanctified, or blameless in God's sight—comes from His work in us. Our role is to gain knowledge about how God works and then let that knowledge change the way we think.

YOU ARE NOT YOUR OWN

What will bring about the most change in you is the realization that you truly are not your own. The apostle Paul writes:

> *Do you not know that your body is the temple of the Holy Spirit who is in you, whom you have from God, and you are not your own? For you were bought at a price; therefore glorify God in your body and in your spirit, which are God's.*
>
> 1 CORINTHIANS 6:19-20

Allow this truth to seep into your heart so that it becomes what you believe. Go beyond surface knowledge to a deep understanding about who you are.

You are a precious pearl in God's eyes. You were created intentionally, with great precision and purpose. Your Father loves you so much that He gave His greatest gift so you could be reconciled into His family. You are chosen. You are valued. You are prized. And you are His! You are His treasured gem, and you are His dwelling place, His home, His abode. You are the temple of the Most High God, not made with the hands of men but instead fashioned by the supreme Architect—your Creator.

With this insight, you can now begin to understand the great value of your physical body. In the same way that God carefully designed the Tabernacle in the Wilderness, He also designed your body. It takes only a little study to get a glimpse of the stunning artistry He used when He made all your parts to work together so you can be strong and have vibrant health.

The Tabernacle contained the Most Holy Place where God met with the high priest. Now we have our own High Priest, the risen Lord, who sits at the right hand of the Father and speaks to Him on our behalf. The apostle John highlighted this when he wrote:

> *My little children, these things I write to you, so that*
> *you may not sin. And if anyone sins, we have an*
> *Advocate with the Father, Jesus Christ the righteous.*

And He Himself is the propitiation for our sins, and not
for ours only but also for the whole world.

Now by this we know that we know Him, if we keep
His commandments. He who says, "I know Him," and
does not keep His commandments, is a liar, and the
truth is not in him. But whoever keeps His word, truly
the love of God is perfected in him. By this we know
that we are in Him. He who says he abides in Him
ought himself also to walk just as He walked.

1 JOHN 2:1-6

As we discussed earlier, when God designed His Tabernacle in the Wilderness, He also gave clear instructions
about its care. He positioned Aaron and his descendants to
be the caretakers of His dwelling place. While Aaron wasn't
perfect, he accepted this position with honor and reverence
to God. He performed his duties with care, diligence, and
responsibility. He protected the Tabernacle and treated it as
the holy place of habitation that it was. He allowed nothing
to defile it because it was not his. It was the dwelling place
of the Most High, designed so God could be in the midst
of His people.

Now God has given you this same responsibility. You are
the caretaker of your body—the temple that God bought
with a price. My hope is that you will embrace these truths
and allow them to be your reason—your incentive—to make
the changes required to be in the best condition, one fitting
for the home of God. Allow the truth about who you are to
be what fuels your commitment to change—and what sets

you free from the bondages of unhealthy eating habits, over-consumption, and poor nutrition.

As you enter into this time of extended prayer and fasting, I encourage you to use your study time to meditate on these truths until they guide your actions. Psalm 119 says, "Your word is a lamp to my feet and a light to my path. . . . Direct my steps by Your word, and let no iniquity have dominion over me" (verses 105 and 133). Let the Scriptures you read in this book and on your own direct you to renewed life.

Throughout the coming chapters you will learn more about what God wants for you and your health, along with proven principles for a healthy lifestyle that will lead to weight loss and increased energy and vitality. But here is the most powerful part of this approach to improved health: You are changing from the inside out. You are changing what you believe. It's this kind of change that renews your thinking and affects your actions—and that in turn leads to the transformation you desire.

WEIGHT LOSS SUCCESS TIP

You've just learned some powerful truths about God, you, and your body. Take a couple of minutes and write a short message to your Creator about your desire to fulfill your role as caretaker of the temple He has entrusted to your care. This would be a good time to commit to the Daniel Fast guidelines and open your heart to learning from the Lord about developing a lifestyle of health and well-being.

CHAPTER 4

Your Body Image and Who You Are in Christ

God's Idea of Beauty

IN THE LAST CHAPTER we looked at scriptural principles for how we should view our bodies—as God's dwelling place, and as His, not our own. Those principles should inform all the choices we make about our health and eating. But we don't live in a vacuum, and our culture tells us very different things about how we should treat our bodies and what makes them worthwhile. In this chapter we'll take a look at how we can counter those cultural messages and remember our true identity. It begins with a powerful tool God constructed in us that we can use for our good: our imagination.

According to *Merriam-Webster*, imagination is "the ability to imagine things that are not real: the ability to form a picture in your mind of something that you have not seen or experienced; the ability to think of new things; something that only exists or happens in your mind."

You and I have the ability to paint a picture in our mind, and this creative process is what helps us look into the future and hope for something beyond our present reality. Our imagination gets us out of the here and now and allows us to picture ourselves in a new scene or a different circumstance.

Our imagination keeps us thinking in pictures, rather than in words. If you hear the word *dog*, an image of a four-legged creature shows up in your mind—not the word. If you hear *black dog*, the image may change. If you then hear *barking black dog*, the picture created by your imagination changes once again.

The imagination is the literary tool that novelists, lyricists, and even psalmists use to paint word pictures so you can "see" what they are describing. Here we observe the great impact of imagery through the written word of the psalmist:

> *He will cover you with his feathers.*
> *He will shelter you with his wings.*
> *His faithful promises are your armor and protection.*
> PSALM 91:4, NLT

We read these words and a picture comes to mind as we imagine being weak, yet safe and secure. We may imagine being wrapped in the protective arms of a strong and loving father, or perhaps safe in a place hidden away from peril. The Scriptures are full of imagery.

Remember the story Jesus told about the Prodigal Son? He asked his father for his inheritance and then promptly squandered it all. Penniless, he decided to come home and throw himself on his father's mercy. As you read the biblical account of the Prodigal Son returning home, try to visualize the scene and see the love, forgiveness, and acceptance exhibited by the father:

> *[The prodigal son] arose and came to his father. But when he was still a great way off, his father saw him and had compassion, and ran and fell on his neck and kissed him. And the son said to him, "Father, I have sinned against heaven and in your sight, and am no longer worthy to be called your son."*
>
> *But the father said to his servants, "Bring out the best robe and put it on him, and put a ring on his hand and sandals on his feet. And bring the fatted calf here and kill it, and let us eat and be merry; for this my son was dead and is alive again; he was lost and is found." And they began to be merry.*
>
> LUKE 15:20-24

Our mind's eye can see the shame-ridden son making his way back home, hoping for even the lowest level of assistance from his father. When his father sees him, he immediately rushes toward the boy he loves so very much and welcomes him back into his arms. As we meditate on this scene and the allegory of how our heavenly Father longs for reconciliation with any who are separated from Him, our own hearts are filled with deep emotion. That triggers understanding and belief about our Lord and His character.

Our imaginations are powerful. They create pictures in our minds that then move us emotionally and spark attitudes, feelings, and beliefs. Beliefs are what fuel our choices and our actions. Again, we see God's wisdom in His instructions to us: "Guard your heart more than anything else, because the source of your life flows from it" (Proverbs 4:23, GW).

THE PICTURES IN OUR MINDS

The images we capture in our minds have a significant impact on the way we think about ourselves—and specifically, the way we feel about the appearance of our physical body. Today, the average American sees more than three thousand advertisements every day (up to five thousand for city dwellers, according to the market research firm Yankelovich).[1] Many of these ads include pictures as well as spoken messages about how we should look. We may not even realize the effect these images have on us. However, the messages enter our minds through our eyes and ears, and unless a stronger truth counters them, they can become truth for us.

The flow of "doctored" images pouring from the airwaves affects people, especially girls and women. That's because even unknowingly, the images we see on television, on computer screens, or in magazines get imprinted on our minds. The next time we look in the mirror and see our reflection, an insidious conversation may take place inside our brains. *Oh, look at that. I'm not very pretty. My legs are too short. My thighs are too big. My hair is too thin. I'm too old. I'm too fat. I'm not very good.* Experts in the field call this "social comparison." The media presents an idealized body image, they say, and so girls and women often fall into the snare of comparing themselves with sociocultural standards of feminine beauty. The consequences are feeling poorly about who you are as a person.

My heart breaks for girls growing up in this age who get caught in the cycle of comparing themselves with these false images of beauty. A recent British study found that 34 percent of girls and 21 percent of boys were upset about weight and body shape. The study also revealed that girls ages 13 and 15 were more than twice as likely as boys of the same age to be "extremely worried" about gaining weight or getting fat.[2] The concern wasn't about their health and what extra pounds might signal about what was happening to their internal organs and body systems. Instead, these youngsters were worried about how they looked to others and how their bodies compared with the ideal image of beauty. Sadly, these feelings, unchecked by truth, can lead to serious consequences, including low self-worth, eating disorders, and even suicide.

The problem doesn't end when we grow up! We carry the deceptions of body image into adult life as we compare ourselves with how others look. We concern ourselves with how others will judge our appearance, and we look into the mirror to receive the visual report about how we measure up to the images we still have imprinted on our minds. Again, if not corrected, the results can be harsh. Consider this statement from the National Eating Disorder Association (NEDA), headquartered in New York City:

In the United States, 20 million women and 10 million men suffer from a clinically significant eating disorder at some time in their life, including anorexia nervosa, bulimia nervosa, binge eating

disorder, or an eating disorder not otherwise specified
(EDNOS). . . . For various reasons, many cases
are likely not to be reported. In addition, many
individuals struggle with body dissatisfaction and
sub-clinical disordered eating attitudes and behaviors,
and the best-known contributor to the development
of anorexia nervosa and bulimia nervosa is body
dissatisfaction. . . . By age 6, girls especially start to
express concerns about their own weight or shape.
40-60% of elementary school girls (ages 6-12) are
concerned about their weight or about becoming too
fat. This concern endures through life.[3]

Body image, our emotions, media pictures of fabricated
beauty, and the lack of exposure to God's truth all contribute to a very real crisis of the soul for millions of girls, boys,
women, and men.

There is something you can do about it for yourself and
for those you can influence. Let's look again at this powerful
and unchanging truth from God's Word:

*I beseech you therefore, brethren, by the mercies of God,
that you present your bodies a living sacrifice, holy,
acceptable to God, which is your reasonable service. And
do not be conformed to this world, but be transformed
by the renewing of your mind, that you may prove what
is that good and acceptable and perfect will of God.*
ROMANS 12:1-2

Accepting what the world has to say about beauty and body image is one way we become "conformed to this world." We can see the destruction this way of thinking can cause as we consider how we feel about our bodies and even how we may judge others. But take heed! We have the ability to change, to heal, and to get on the right path. The apostle Paul wrote these encouraging words: "There is therefore now no condemnation to those who are in Christ Jesus, who do not walk according to the flesh, but according to the Spirit" (Romans 8:1).

We can renew our minds to the truth of God, our Creator, and then with practice and focus we can walk according to the Spirit. We can experience what it means for God's truth to free us from the deceitfulness of cultural images of beauty. And instead of getting approval about how we look from people, we can see ourselves for who we are (the temple of God's Holy Spirit). We can acknowledge that each and every person was created in the image of God with a different standard for beauty.

I like the way the Living Bible paints a word picture for us:

You made all the delicate, inner parts of my body and knit them together in my mother's womb. Thank you for making me so wonderfully complex! It is amazing to think about. Your workmanship is marvelous—and how well I know it. You were there while I was being formed in utter seclusion!

Psalm 139:13-15, TLB

Our God is a masterful Designer, and we do well when we understand that He made us on purpose. He is the Potter and we are the clay. Every person was made as He desired, and His definition of beauty is far different from what we find in our society.

A NEW WAY OF THINKING

Before we trash fashion and mirrors, let's look at them in a positive light. Looking clean, put together, and even fashionable is okay! When we read about wardrobes in the Scriptures, we often find clothing made of fine fabrics and women being adorned with jewels. In Ezekiel we can see how God used the imagery of clothing and jewelry to express His great love and care for Jerusalem:

> *I gave you expensive clothing of fine linen and silk, beautifully embroidered, and sandals made of fine goatskin leather. I gave you lovely jewelry, bracelets, beautiful necklaces, a ring for your nose, earrings for your ears, and a lovely crown for your head. And so you were adorned with gold and silver. Your clothes were made of fine linen and costly fabric and were beautifully embroidered. You ate the finest foods— choice flour, honey, and olive oil—and became more beautiful than ever. You looked like a queen, and so you were! Your fame soon spread throughout the world because of your beauty. I dressed you in my splendor and perfected your beauty, says the Sovereign LORD.*
> EZEKIEL 16:10-14, NLT

When we gaze at a sunset or regard the beauty of snow-covered peaks against a brilliant blue sky, we're seeing how our Creator adorned the earth and made it beautiful. Beauty is not a bad thing, and neither is fashion or looking at ourselves in a mirror. The tipping point is when pride enters. Even in the example above, when God "dressed" Jerusalem beautifully, we only need to continue reading to see the dark side of Jerusalem's prideful response:

> *But you thought your fame and beauty were your own.*
> *So you gave yourself as a prostitute to every man who*
> *came along. Your beauty was theirs for the asking. You*
> *used the lovely things I gave you to make shrines for*
> *idols, where you played the prostitute. Unbelievable!*
> *How could such a thing ever happen? You took the*
> *very jewels and gold and silver ornaments I had given*
> *you and made statues of men and worshiped them.*
> *This is adultery against me! You used the beautifully*
> *embroidered clothes I gave you to dress your idols. Then*
> *you used my special oil and my incense to worship them.*
> *Imagine it! You set before them as a sacrifice the choice*
> *flour, olive oil, and honey I had given you, says the*
> *Sovereign LORD.*
>
> EZEKIEL 16:15-19, NLT

God creates only what is good. When pride contaminates His creation, all is spoiled, and beauty becomes ugliness. But when we think of ourselves as human beings created in the image of God and intentionally made, we can indeed see beauty in ourselves. That's not because of our definition of beauty, but because of His. Acknowledging such beauty is not prideful, because it's not something we have manufactured. Our beauty comes from God Himself and the care He put into creating us.

When God designed the Tabernacle in the Wilderness, He used superior materials, including gold, silver, and bronze. He ordered tapestries woven with fine linen and vibrant colors of blue, purple, and scarlet. In Revelation 21:21, we learn of heaven's adornments: "The twelve gates were twelve pearls: each individual gate was of one pearl. And the street of the city was pure gold, like transparent glass." God clearly values beauty. However, the beauty is by His definition and not the world's. His beauty is grounded in love, virtue, and righteousness rather than ego, pride, and self.

A HOLY IMAGE

When God created you, it was in His image. In the same way He designed the Tabernacle in the Wilderness with unique features and artfulness, He created you with precision and specific intention.

Please, get this truth into your heart: God lovingly created you on purpose, and He is molding you into exactly who He wants you to be. Of course we live in a fallen world, and we see the effects of that on our bodies, souls, and spirits. Yet what God created is good, as we see in Genesis 1:31: "Then God saw everything that He had made, and indeed it was very good."

The image our Lord wants us to embrace, the mirror

He wants us to use, is His image of us. Not the world's standards. Not the pictures on television. Not the doctored photos in magazines. The truth of who you are is the perfectly created and beautiful human being that your Creator made.

I realize that this concept will not immediately change people's minds and attitudes about themselves. We need to spend time with this reality and allow God's truth about us to change our perceptions. As you experience these twenty-one days of extended prayer and fasting, my hope is that each day you will remind yourself of this truth from God's Word:

For You formed my inward parts;
You covered me in my mother's womb.
I will praise You, for I am fearfully and wonderfully
          made;
Marvelous are Your works,
And that my soul knows very well.
My frame was not hidden from You,
When I was made in secret,
And skillfully wrought in the lowest parts of the earth.
Your eyes saw my substance, being yet unformed.
And in Your book they all were written,
The days fashioned for me,
When as yet there were none of them.

How precious also are Your thoughts to me, O God!
How great is the sum of them!

> *If I should count them, they would be more in number*
> *than the sand;*
> *When I awake, I am still with You.*
>
> PSALM 139:13-18

God's truth is the image we want to gaze upon. And when we look into the "mirror" of who He created us to be, the real us will be reflected back.

WEIGHT LOSS SUCCESS TIP

A well-nourished and adequately hydrated body takes on a healthy glow. This is the type of beauty planned by God. Add in the light of Christ shining through you—including love, joy, and a peaceful countenance—and you have everything you need for beauty.

So often we crave more when what we have is enough. Today, with every meal and glass of water, pause to be thankful for how beautifully God is meeting your daily needs in both body and soul. How does this reflection change your habits and your approach to eating?

CHAPTER 5

Resetting Your Body for Weight Loss and Health

Physical Benefits of the Daniel Fast

WE'VE JUST ESTABLISHED THE SPIRITUAL TRUTHS that are the foundation for caring for our bodies well. Our ultimate incentive for pursuing health is that our bodies are temples of the Holy Spirit, and we want to treat them with the care and respect they deserve. But there are physical incentives as well. In this chapter we'll look at how the Daniel Fast can improve some common health issues and lead you to a stronger, healthier body.

Our bodies are constantly active. Every second they are dynamically engaged in carrying out the processes needed for our health. Even now as you read these words, your cardiovascular system is transporting nutrients, oxygen, carbon dioxide, hormones, and blood cells to and from parts of the body to nourish it, help fight diseases, stabilize your body temperature, and encourage growth. Your lungs provide you with the oxygen you need to live while also removing carbon dioxide before it can reach hazardous levels. Your digestive system is breaking down the food you've consumed into smaller and smaller components, which can be absorbed into your body for sustenance.

Complex. Stunning. Amazing. Elegant. All of these words describe our Creator's intricate and purposeful design for the human body. He constructed every part of it to work perfectly, and He also designed foods that would be the perfect match, providing just what your body needs.

Many times we have unknowingly, or perhaps even out of rebellion, chosen foods and developed habits that don't support good health. When these unhealthy behaviors continue over time, they can bring harm to the perfect systems God created. For example, type 2 diabetes is usually caused by eating too much of the wrong kinds of food. Heart disease is often triggered by the same thing, as is high blood pressure. The list goes on and on. When we continually consume foods that are not good for our bodies, at some point our bodies break down. Consequently, disease and infirmities set in, and then we encounter serious health problems.

Here is the really great thing about starting your journey into a healthy lifestyle with the Daniel Fast: During your twenty-one-day fasting experience, your body will undergo a wall-to-wall renovation. It all happens because of the foods you eat and the water you drink, along with drenching yourself in prayer and meditation.

The Daniel Fast—with its emphasis on natural foods and lots of vegetables and fruits—is a healthy and nutrient-rich way of eating. And since the only beverage on the Daniel

Fast is water, your body will be constantly flushed with liquid cleanser! Day by day, as you give your body clean and wholesome foods and drink plenty of water, it will be purged of toxins. Imbalances in your system will come into harmony, and your body will begin resetting itself into the healthy temple God intended. Not only will you begin to give your body the foods it needs so it can operate properly, but as you submit more of who you are to the Lord and allow Him to fill your needs, you will also find that overeating goes away and the pounds begin to vanish.

FOUNDATION OF SUBMISSION

The key to getting these powerful renovation processes started is your decision to submit yourself—your spirit, soul, and body—to your Creator. According to the *Merriam-Webster Dictionary*, submission is "the state of being obedient: the act of accepting the authority or control of someone else; the condition of being submissive, humble, or compliant; an act of submitting to the authority or control of another."

Each person beginning the Daniel Fast must ask, "Am I willing to submit myself to what I think the Lord is calling me to do?" That is not a light question, and we should not answer without deep consideration. When we say, "Yes," to the Lord, we are saying, "I will put myself and my desires aside. I will put my trust in You. I humbly agree to comply with the fasting principles for this spiritual experience."

Don't be surprised if you sense a stirring inside. You may feel a little anxious. A little uneasy. Even a little fearful. That is totally normal. It happens because you are stepping into a real place with your Lord. You are entering into the fast. You are making a commitment to Him to leave any unhealthy wants and desires outside and step into a new experience that He directs.

When you choose the way of the Lord, you also open yourself to His tools and His help. Part of that comes by opening your heart to His truths as He speaks to you through His Word. Then as you meditate on those truths, you allow yourself to "be transformed by the renewing of your mind, that you may prove what is that good and acceptable and perfect will of God" (Romans 12:2).

This is part of the mystery of our faith. As followers of Jesus Christ, we have the Holy Spirit working within us. His Spirit connects with our spirit. We gain revelation, power, and renewal. This is the internal restoration that is made possible through Jesus.

> *The Spirit of the LORD is upon Me,*
> *Because He has anointed Me*
> *To preach the gospel to the poor;*
> *He has sent Me to heal the brokenhearted,*
> *To proclaim liberty to the captives*
> *And recovery of sight to the blind,*
> *To set at liberty those who are oppressed.*
> LUKE 4:18

When you submit your heart to the heart of God, then you are "given to know the mystery of the kingdom of God" (Mark 4:11). That privilege comes through your sincere agreement to put yourself under the authority and care of your Father and then allow Him to reveal His truths to your heart so they can change the way you live.

When you commit yourself to submitting to God, you unleash a power that is not your own. Instead, it's the power of the Lord working in you. And when you couple this interior action of the heart with the wise food choices included in the Daniel Fast eating plan, the results are more than you could ever accomplish on your own.

By giving up your will to God's, you will soon see the demise of cravings for foods that you thought you could never go without. You will notice a surge of empowerment. And as you continue on this path, you will gain a new strength found only as you walk in the light of God's ways. This mystery of our faith is available to us, yet we can only experience it when we submit ourselves to the Lord and allow Him to work through us.

OUT WITH THE OLD—DETOXING YOUR BODY

As I hope you've come to understand, the Daniel Fast is first a spiritual experience. To gain the best results for your whole self—your spirit, soul, and body—you'll want to keep the spiritual focus at the forefront. But meanwhile, as you draw nearer to God; as you gain understanding about who and what you are; and as you fast, meaning you restrict food for a spiritual purpose, your body will undergo a certain level of detox.

The word *detox* has two parts. *De* means "to separate from," and *tox* is derived from the word *toxin*, which means "poison." So when your body is in detox, it is going away from or separating from the poisons that have accumulated in it. Our bodies become toxic from a multitude of sources, including the foods we eat and the beverages we drink. Toxins also exist in cosmetics, lotions, soaps, cleaners, and the air.

You have probably heard of more radical ways to detox your body solely for health purposes. Those usually include complete abstinence from food for a period of time and can be coupled with medical procedures. The Daniel Fast, by contrast, contributes to detox in three primary ways. First, you will not be consuming chemicals that are included in packaged foods. Second, you will eat only nourishing foods that allow your body to more easily execute its own detox functions. And third, you will drink only water as your beverage, which naturally serves as the most powerful detox agent.

If eating clean foods—whole foods that are free of chemicals and additives—is new to you, then you may experience some physical discomfort on the first few days of your fast. To avoid these symptoms, I strongly encourage you to prepare your body for the Daniel Fast (see chapter 2).

Let's take a look at three of the most beneficial aspects of the Daniel Fast eating plan: consuming more fiber, consuming less sugar, and drinking lots of water.

WHY FIBER IS ESSENTIAL FOR GOOD HEALTH

The Daniel Fast eating plan includes a substantial amount of fiber, and your digestive system may not be accustomed to the increased amount. The discomfort is giving you a message that you need to continually provide adequate fiber in your menus to keep your body functioning in optimum health.

Fiber comes from the portion of plants—including fruits, vegetables, and whole grains—that the digestive enzymes in your system cannot break down. This part of the food is not wasted, however. Fiber fulfills an essential function and maintains optimal health—another example of God's amazing wisdom when He created us.

Fiber adds bulk and moisture for the body's elimination and prevents constipation. It also cleans out your intestines to keep your digestive system in good working order. Plus, when you have adequate fiber in your system, you feel full and satisfied, which aids in weight loss.

Part of the fiber (called soluble fiber) turns into a gel-like substance while it's in the intestine. This fiber acts like a sponge and can help reduce LDL cholesterol, which is a waxy substance created in the liver. LDL molecules travel through the bloodstream to cells throughout the body that use the cholesterol to produce hormones and provide structure to cell membranes. That's all essential for good health. Problems arise when too much cholesterol in our body increases the LDL levels, causing the excess waxy substance to accumulate in our blood vessels. This buildup promotes atherosclerosis, the formation of plaque and hardening of the arteries, which leads to heart disease. Soluble fiber found in oatmeal, beans, peas, and some fruits helps prevent this problem.

Let's take a look at what is happening during the digestive process. First, your liver produces and processes cholesterol, using it to make bile acids that are stored in your gallbladder. When you eat fat, the gallbladder sends the bile into your intestines, where the bile acids break apart the fat molecules so the fat and fat-soluble vitamins can be used for your health. Your body then reabsorbs any leftover bile, about 95 percent of what was excreted, and sends it back into the bloodstream. It's returned to the liver and back to the gallbladder, which will re-excrete the bile acids the next time they're needed.

When adequate fiber is present in your intestine, it binds to the bile acids and removes them from your body through elimination. This decreases the amount of bile recirculated, which in turn means that your liver needs to use more cholesterol to produce more bile acids. The end result is that there isn't as much cholesterol in your body to make LDL, reducing your risk of heart disease.

The Daniel Fast eating plan includes the very foods your body needs for adequate fiber: fruits, vegetables, legumes, and whole grains. You are giving your body what it needs to operate as God intended. This is why many people with high cholesterol find their levels moving into healthy ranges in just twenty-one days without medication and only with food.

AVOIDING EXCESS SUGAR

Your body may need more of some nutrients, such as fiber. It also most likely needs much less of another food—sugar, especially the highly processed variety found in sugar bowls, desserts, pastries, cereals, and in a surprising number of processed foods.

Health experts report that American adults consume an average of more than 150 pounds of sugar each year.[1] Imagine that! Can you see a five-pound bag of sugar in your mind's eye? Now imagine thirty five-pound bags stacked on your dining table. That's a lot of sugar going through your system every year.

Sadly, increased sugar consumption is a trend moving in the wrong direction. Almost two hundred years ago, the average American consumed 45 grams of sugar every five days. By 2012, that number had increased to 765 grams.[2] Get this: These days the typical teenage boy consumes more than 34 teaspoons of sugar each day![3] Most is what is called "refined sugar" and comes from cane sugar, beet sugar, corn syrup, and corn sugar. Much of that is consumed in the sodas many teens—and adults—drink throughout the day.

God did not create our bodies to eat this way. What happens when we do?

Here is what it looks like when sugar is refined:

The natural sugar that is stored in the cane stalk or beet root is separated from the rest of the plant material. For sugar cane, this is accomplished by:

- Grinding the cane to extract the juice;
- Boiling the juice until the syrup thickens and crystallizes;
- Spinning the crystals in a centrifuge to produce raw sugar;
- Shipping the raw sugar to a refinery, where it is

- Washed and filtered to remove remaining non-sugar ingredients and color; and
- Crystallized, dried, and packaged.

Beet sugar processing is similar, but it is done in one continuous process without the raw sugar stage. The sugar beets are washed, sliced, and soaked in hot water to separate the sugar-containing juice from the beet fiber. The sugar-laden juice is purified, filtered, concentrated, and dried in a series of steps similar to sugar cane processing.[4]

You might be surprised by what gives refined sugar its pure white color. An article from the Vegetarian Resource Group states,

The average consumer's love affair with white, sweet foods prompted the sugar industry to develop a sugar refining process that would yield "pure" white crystals. Hundreds of years ago, sugar refiners discovered that bone char from cattle worked well as a whitening filter, and this practice is now the industry standard.[5]

Whether "raw" or refined, sugar has no nutritional value and leads to empty calories. An article from Mayo Clinic states, "Despite what you may have heard, there's no nutritional advantage for honey, brown sugar, fruit juice concentrate or other types of sugar over white sugar."[6]

Here's the good news: When people eat sugar, their blood

sugar levels rise and the pancreas produces insulin. Insulin is a hormone that tells your cells to absorb the blood sugar so it can be used for energy. As the cells absorb the blood sugar, levels in the bloodstream begin to fall. This action then triggers the pancreas to start making glucagon, a hormone that tells the liver to start releasing stored sugar. This interchange makes sure that the cells throughout your body, and especially in your brain, have a steady supply of blood sugar, giving them the energy they need.

Now for the bad news: When too much sugar is consumed (remember that image of thirty five-pound bags of sugar stacked on your dining table), your pancreas is not able to keep up with the demand for insulin. In addition, your cells are not able to keep up with the load and eventually start to shut down. This is called "insulin resistance" and is often the precursor to type 2 diabetes. A person with diabetes will have fluctuating blood sugars, which can eventually lead to blindness, kidney failure, cardiovascular disease, nerve damage, and amputation of feet and legs.

God's Way

Our bodies need sugar—but our Creator designed our bodies to use the natural sugar in foods to make energy so we can live, work, and do what we need to do. He created foods to meet this need. When these whole foods are consumed, the digestion process takes time, allowing the natural sugars to be released slowly into the bloodstream. Our bodies are able to keep up with the demand to process the sugars, and they receive what we need for good health.

Optimal whole foods are made up of complex carbo-hydrates because of their cell structure components. Many complex-carbohydrate foods contain fiber, vitamins, and minerals, and they take longer for the body to digest.

Simple carbohydrate foods, on the other hand, are much easier to digest and send the sugar into the bloodstream quickly, causing sugar spikes and wreaking havoc on your body. Eating many of these simple carbohydrate foods, also called high-glycemic foods, can lead to an increased risk of type 2 diabetes, heart disease, mood swings, fatigue, and weight gain. Simple carbohydrate foods are refined or highly processed, including sugar, baked goods made with white flour, white rice, white-flour pasta, pastries, candy, and sodas.

The Daniel Fast Way

The Daniel Fast eating plan includes no refined grains (only whole grains) and no added sweeteners. Of course, it's impos-sible to avoid all sugars, as just about every food includes some natural sugar. God planned it that way. However, He also intended for these foods to stay intact rather than be processed so much that all the beneficial parts are removed.

You will discover while you are on the Daniel Fast that many manufacturers of packaged foods add refined sugar to their recipes, boosting the amount of sugar the average per-son consumes each year. You will get in the habit of reading the list of ingredients on food labels to discover whether the product complies with the Daniel Fast guidelines. This is a habit you will want to use after the fast as you continue on your path toward a lifestyle of health.

LIVING WATER: MAINTAINING HYDRATION IN OUR SPIRIT AND SOUL

Our spirit, soul, and body all need adequate water for good health. Jesus taught the Samaritan woman at the well about the essential water we need for our inner life: "If you knew the gift of God, and who it is who says to you, 'Give Me a drink,' you would have asked Him, and He would have given you living water" (John 4:10).

To remain strong in our faith, we need to have a constant flow of the living water from God's Word entering into our spirit. When we have this continuous flow of His truth, we are able to live the faith-driven life we are called to and be the witnesses of God's love and grace that He wants us to be. Through our actions, we serve as examples for others to see. Jesus told His disciples, "He who believes in Me, as the Scripture has said, out of his heart will flow rivers of living water" (John 7:38).

Our soul, that mental and emotional part of our being, also needs to drink from good and life-giving sources. The Bible teaches us a fundamental truth about our beings in this familiar verse: "For as he thinketh in his heart, so is he" (Proverbs 23:7, KJV). If we fully embrace that truth, we will be careful about what we allow to enter into our thinking.

Proverbs 4:23 says, "Keep your heart with all diligence, for out of it spring the issues of life." I often imagine my mind as a tall glass of water sitting on a table. If I don't do anything to guard the glass, the water will evaporate into the elements and may even accumulate dust and unpleasant particles from the surrounding atmosphere. The glass is replenished by what I pour into it, and I have the choice about what will go in. Will it be life-giving knowledge, entertainment, and images? Or will it be content that pulls me down or contaminates the water in the glass? The choice is mine. I try to always choose good, clean water for my soul that will stimulate growth, goodness, and godliness.

The apostle Paul spoke to this important part of our lives in one of my favorite passages when he taught about choosing what to set our minds on:

> *Finally, brethren, whatever things are true,*
> *whatever things are noble, whatever things are*
> *just, whatever things are pure, whatever things*
> *are lovely, whatever things are of good report, if there*
> *is any virtue and if there is anything praiseworthy—*
> *meditate on these things.*
>
> Philippians 4:8

"Meditate on these things," teaches the apostle. Think about what is good and right and helpful. This is the water we want to pour into our souls so that we can have the life we want and the life our Lord wants for us. I love this image from the prophet Jeremiah:

> *Blessed is the man who trusts in the LORD,*
> *And whose hope is the LORD.*
> *For he shall be like a tree planted by the waters,*
> *Which spreads out its roots by the river,*
> *And will not fear when heat comes;*

But its leaf will be green,
And will not be anxious in the year of drought,
Nor will cease from yielding fruit.

JEREMIAH 17:7-8

I want to be like a tree planted by the water—someone who continually has access to God's life-giving, refreshing presence. I want to intentionally fill my soul with good, clean, and nourishing water.

The Physical Body

Our physical bodies also depend on a constant flow of good, clean, and nourishing water. Most people are surprised to learn that water makes up more than half of your body weight. Every part of your body, including its cells, tissue, and organs, needs water to function properly. Sixty percent of your body is made up of water. Your muscles are 75 percent water, and your brain is 85 percent water! Water is to our bodies like oil to a machine.[7]

Health experts find that up to 75 percent of all American adults drink far less water than the body requires and therefore are in a chronic state of dehydration. No wonder we have achy joints and sore muscles. In a news article quoting Mary Grace Webb, Assistant Director for Clinical Nutrition at New York Hospital, we read,

> "The human body is so unique that it will say
> 'I want water' in food, in any way, shape or form,"
> Webb said. "People just think that when they start

to get a little weak or they have a headache, they need to eat something, but most often they need to drink."

Water is necessary for the body to digest and absorb vitamins and nutrients. It's also key to proper digestion; it detoxifies the liver and kidneys, and carries waste away, Webb said.

"If your urine becomes darkly colored . . . , we're dehydrated. The urine should be light, straw colored," Webb explained.[8]

Over time, not being adequately hydrated can contribute to a variety of health complications, including joint pain, weight gain, headaches, ulcers, high blood pressure, kidney disease, and fatigue.

Water on Your Daniel Fast

The Daniel Fast serves as an excellent opportunity to develop the habit of drinking adequate amounts of water. We'll talk more about this later in the book, but simply put, I encourage people to drink four tall glasses or bottles of water each day. That's just 16 ounces in each glass, and you can spread them throughout the day to make sure you stay hydrated.

When you adopt this habit, you will soon see multiple health benefits, including more energy, less joint pain, and weight loss because you will feel fuller and not desire as much food.

The Daniel Fast provides an eating plan that gives your body what it yearns for to operate at optimum health. During this twenty-one-day period of eating vitamin-rich and nutritious whole foods, you are cleansing your body of the toxins that have accumulated, plus you are resetting your systems so that they can function optimally and improve your health.

The great news is that when you stay within the Daniel Fast guidelines, you don't have to go to a lot of extra effort to figure out how to give your body what it needs for healing and good health. Vegetables, fruits, and whole grains all provide the fiber your body needs to function properly. Cutting out refined sugars and consuming only foods with naturally occurring sugars eliminates the blood-sugar spikes that cause hunger pangs and cravings. And drinking plenty of water provides the cleansing liquid to keep your body operating in good health. My hope is that even when you are finished with the twenty-one-day fast, you will maintain these good habits and reap the benefits for the rest of your life. That's what developing a lifestyle of health is all about.

WEIGHT LOSS SUCCESS TIP

One of the best changes you can develop is to make sure you have nutritious foods readily available in your home, workplace, and even your car. Imagine three healthy food items you enjoy that you can keep on hand during your Daniel Fast. Stock up on these foods. Then when you want a snack, you already know what to eat—and it's right there waiting for you!

CHAPTER 6

Flesh, Sit Down! You Are Out of Order

Dealing with Physical and Spiritual Temptation

WE ALL KNOW we should be eating fewer processed foods and refined sugars, but let's be honest: Sometimes we really, really want them. In this chapter we'll talk about how to deal with our physical cravings, both on the fast and afterward. We'll also go beyond that. The truth is, cravings are not just a physical problem. When we want something and think we have to have it, we're really dealing with a spiritual battle against the flesh, or our sinful nature. Our inability to say no to potato chips is just a symptom of a bigger issue.

CRAVINGS, BEGONE

Our problem with cravings is often connected to the foods we consume. When we eat processed, sugar-laden foods, we send our bodies on a roller coaster of steep spikes, followed by abrupt descents. Highs and lows. Ups and downs. And when we do that, we set ourselves up for cravings, hunger pangs, and even major mood swings.

Also, when we give our bodies "empty calories"—high in sugar but low in or almost devoid of nutrients—our bodies start screaming for goodness. Empty calories supply food energy but minimal nutrition, and when the body receives an abundance of this kind of food energy, it stores the excess as fat. The processes required tax the body's working systems in a way that can cause malfunction and major breakdowns.

Meanwhile, the body remains in want of what it really needs to operate as it was designed, so it starts talking to us! The clamorings for vitamins, minerals, and other essential elements come in the form of hunger. When our minds are not in tune with what our physical body really needs and instead we respond to the call for help with more empty calories, the body can only react. More highs and lows. More ups and downs. More cravings. The roller coaster in this unhealthy carnival of consumption continues, and the result is a broken-down system, poor health, and weight gain. This disrepair, neglect, and brokenness provoke additional damage that can be irreversible, such as the health consequences associated with diabetes, including blindness and amputation of limbs; cardiovascular disease leading to heart attack and strokes; and even the emotional challenges of food addictions.

Add in dehydration, and you have a recipe for even more havoc. When the body needs water, it sends a subtle signal to your brain—even before you feel thirsty. Unless you are attuned to your body, you will likely read this plea for water as a demand for food. And what do you do when you think your body wants food? You feed it. Sadly, most people who are overweight mistakenly respond with more empty calories, which then incites the roller-coaster cycle, allowing the devastation to continue.

When you feed your body with nutrient-dense foods, which are those included in the Daniel Fast, the cycle stops! Do you get that? The cycle of destruction stops. Your blood sugar remains more stable, you feel satisfied, and you avoid those abrupt increases and drops in energy. And bit by bit, as you continue to give your body what it needs, the hunger pangs and the cravings stop too.

Mix this very real phenomenon with the living water going into your spirit and soul, and you are now on a path that leads to healing, well-being, increased energy, and vitality. You are being realigned with how you are intended to live. Your body starts to shed the stored fat and begins to operate in the way the Designer planned. You start to feel calmer, more balanced, and encouraged. This change comes from the inside out. It's the pathway to transformation and your way to a forever lifestyle of health.

The best offense against cravings is a good defense. Stay nourished by eating three healthy meals and two snacks each day. Stay away from fruits that have a lot of sugar, white potatoes, and other foods that are high on the glycemic index (to learn more, visit www.glycemicindex.com). The key to success is to stay nourished and not let yourself get hungry. When you do this, you will be surprised and pleased by how rarely you are hit with cravings!

CRAVINGS ON THE DANIEL FAST

When you first begin your Daniel Fast, you might experience some cravings. The intensity and length of cravings usually depends on what makes up your typical meals, as well as how well you've prepared your body for the fast by tapering off sugar and processed foods.

I have worked with hundreds of people who know they are addicted to sugar. Sugar addictions can be tough to break, but be of good cheer! It is possible. Yes, you may go through some tough times. If you always have sugar at certain times of day (such as a bowl of ice cream before bed), you may feel deprived or even have a physical sensation of needing the sugar to function well. Some people experience headaches, fatigue, or irritability along with intense cravings. Reading this book and adopting the principles I've shared will measurably reduce your cravings and make it easier for you to resist them.

Don't try to do this all on your own. Pray yourself up! Meditate on God's Word—both the passages shared in these pages and others that are encouraging to you. Allow the Spirit of God within you to help you break the addiction. Take in this truth: You have the option, and His invitation, to ask the Creator of everything for help! Let Jesus be your personal trainer. Let the Holy Spirit be your coach. Use the gifts of helps that come through the Spirit. And soak into the rest that your Lord promises you. Hear His invitation that comes from His heart to yours:

> *Come to Me, all you who labor and are heavy laden,*
> *and I will give you rest. Take My yoke upon you and*

*learn from Me, for I am gentle and lowly in heart, and
you will find rest for your souls. For My yoke is easy
and My burden is light.*

Matthew 11:28-30

If you find yourself laden with the heaviness of food or
sugar addictions, turn to Jesus. If you find yourself strug-
gling to stay away from breads, sodas, or hamburgers, come
to Jesus. If you find yourself weak and tired, come to Jesus.
He has the answers. He wants to help. And He knows what
to do.

Use Your Words

If you sense a craving coming on, don't just go with it.
Instead, pause and speak to that craving! Look at what Jesus
said to his disciples: "Assuredly, I say to you, if you have faith
and do not doubt, you will not only do what was done to the
fig tree, but also if you say to this mountain, 'Be removed
and be cast into the sea,' it will be done" (Matthew 21:21).

Speaking to your body; speaking to cravings; speaking to
mountains—it might all be new to you. But this is the advice
of our Master, so give it a go and don't give up on your first,
second, or even third try. In faith, speak to that craving and
tell it, "Hush!" Then go get a drink of water or a healthy
alternative. Rather than kicking, screaming, and complain-
ing, which actually feeds the craving rather than starves it,
do what parents tell their toddlers to do: "Use your words!"

The Bible teaches us that God created the entire world by
using His words. Hebrews 11:3 says, "By faith we understand

that the worlds were framed by the word of God, so that the things which are seen were not made of things which are visible."

Think about that. Meditate on that truth. Words are powerful, and you can use yours to conquer your flesh. Watch as the cravings start to melt away.

Don't Go Back

Going without sugar and unhealthy foods for the twenty-one days of the Daniel Fast will allow most people to break their addictions. So once you've overcome addictions to food or sugar, don't go back—especially right after you complete your fast. Stick with the principles for staying healthy covered in this book, including the "Ten Habits Practiced by Healthy Individuals" discussed in chapter 7.

You are in the process of developing new "muscle" strength, new habits, and new abilities to withstand food temptation. Give yourself time to deeply embed this new way of eating in your routines and the way you relate to food. Stay strong. Stay on course. Receive and keep the gifts of peace and joy the Lord deposits in your heart as you travel your journey toward a life of health and wellness.

SUBDUING THE FLESH

When we deal with cravings, there's more at stake than just whether or not we eat the chocolate or the french fries. There's a spiritual battle going on too.

I sometimes have what I've labeled "out-of-body experiences." That's not what they really are, but the name fits because during those times I observe myself as if from the outside, taking on the role of the objective investigator. When I discover something about myself that isn't in line with how I know God wants me to be, then I work on making changes.

I remember an occasion when I was hit with a craving for potato chips, which at the time was my number one unhealthy food weakness. I had one of those "Just like Paul" moments: "I don't understand why I act the way I do. I don't do the good I want to do, and I do the evil I hate" (Romans 7:15, ERV). Part of me was saying, "You know those chips aren't good for you, and you know you can't eat just one. So don't start." But another part was saying, "You know how much you like them. You love the saltiness and the crunch. They are so good. Come on! It's okay. Eat the chips."

That's when I had my pseudo out-of-body experience. I looked at what was going on and witnessed the lusts of the flesh trying to sabotage my intentions to eat clean and healthy. I realized the wise part of me, the part of me that is submitted to God, needed to step up and take charge. So the wise Susan said, "Flesh, sit down! You are out of order." It was kind of like telling a child what to do. I was surprised by how this simple act diminished the craving almost instantly.

One of the most valuable lessons we can learn on the Daniel Fast has to do with the internal battle between the Spirit and the flesh. The Bible says, "Walk in the Spirit, and you shall not fulfill the lust of the flesh" (Galatians 5:16). When we submit ourselves to God, we put our flesh— our physical selves, ego, and worldly longings—under His authority. We follow His commands. But oh, can our sinful nature rear its head and fight for its own way! And in today's culture, where the flesh is being tempted and served at almost every turn, it's no wonder that we are in constant battle.

THE POWER OF DECISION

The flesh is not an unbridled force against which we have no control. Reining in the flesh starts with making choices about how we want to behave and what we want for our lives. As followers of Jesus Christ, we are given instructions through Scripture. Our God wants us to live a life that is good, that brings us joy and peace, and that is honoring to Him. He shows us the way, and then it is up to us to choose whether we are willing to follow. God set this choice before the Israelites after He rescued them from slavery in Egypt. The Promised Land lay before them, full of blessings and safety if they only determined to follow God. Moses reviewed the covenant with the people and made this clear to them:

> For this commandment which I command you today
> is not too mysterious for you, nor is it far off. It is not
> in heaven, that you should say, "Who will ascend into
> heaven for us and bring it to us, that we may hear it
> and do it?" Nor is it beyond the sea, that you should say,
> "Who will go over the sea for us and bring it to us, that
> we may hear it and do it?" But the word is very near
> you, in your mouth and in your heart, that you may
> do it.
>
> See, I have set before you today life and good, death
> and evil, in that I command you today to love the

LORD your God, to walk in His ways, and to keep His
commandments, His statutes, and His judgments, that
you may live and multiply; and the LORD your God
will bless you in the land which you go to possess. But if
your heart turns away so that you do not hear, and are
drawn away, and worship other gods and serve them,
I announce to you today that you shall surely perish;
you shall not prolong your days in the land which you
cross over the Jordan to go in and possess. I call heaven
and earth as witnesses today against you, that I have set
before you life and death, blessing and cursing; therefore
choose life, that both you and your descendants may
live; that you may love the LORD your God, that you
may obey His voice, and that you may cling to Him, for
He is your life and the length of your days; and that you
may dwell in the land which the LORD swore to your
fathers, to Abraham, Isaac, and Jacob, to give them.

DEUTERONOMY 30:11-20

Our God is so good. In my own paraphrase of this passage, He is saying, "This isn't a hard choice. The answer isn't far away. It's right here in front of you—plus, I'm telling you the right answer! If you want a great future for yourself and for your family, choose life by doing what I tell you to do."

The choice is ours, every day, every hour. Do we want to walk in the Spirit, in the path directed by our Lord? Or do we want to do things our own way and see how it goes? Do we want to follow the ways of the flesh, which are trained by the world? Or do we want to submit ourselves—which means admitting that we don't know it all—and follow the ways of the Lord who does know it all?

This is where the power of making a decision comes in. When we accept Christ as our Savior, we are making the most important decision of our lives. No other choice has more impact or greater consequence. I still remember "the hour I first believed." I was twenty-four years old and preparing for an informal debate about whether Jesus was merely a wise man (my opinion) or if He was instead the Son of God. I had a week to get ready for the debate, and so I started to cram. Every night I would lie in bed and study the Gospels. I needed to learn more about what this book—that's all the Bible was to me at the time—had to say.

As I focused my attention on Jesus and His actions on earth, I could see that He was indeed a man of great wisdom, justice, kindness, and love. And then about four nights into my study, it happened. I can still remember that internal shift. I took my eyes off the words in the Bible, set the book down on my chest, and just lay there as I realized it was true.

God's Word and His truth penetrated my heart. At that moment, I believed. And while I wasn't yet sure about what that would mean for my future, I did know that I had changed. The decision to believe immediately sparked a new birth inside of me. John 3:16 tells us that the decision to believe moves us from death to life: "For God so loved the world that He gave His only begotten Son, that whoever believes in Him should not perish but have everlasting life."

At that very moment my spirit came alive and the Spirit of God came into my being. Ever since that time I have been on a path to follow the ways of Jesus. I've had my ups and my downs. I've made mistakes, and I've experienced great victories. I thank God that I remain on the path following the teachings of Jesus and continue to grow in His knowledge and love.

Following the ways of the Lord starts with a decision that we will do our best to study, learn, and follow. We submit our way of thinking to God's truth. This act of submission comes from love for our amazing God, who cares so very much for us. But the decision to submit also comes from straight-up smarts! After all, is there any contest about who knows how to live a great life—God or me? God or you? No, we know the answer. Our God knows what is best for us. He says to us, "I call heaven and earth as witnesses today against you, that I have set before you life and death, blessing and cursing; therefore choose life, that both you and your descendants may live" (Deuteronomy 30:19), and He even tells us the best answer: Choose life.

While the decision to follow Christ is the most important choice we'll ever make, it's far from the only important one. As we continue our life journey, we continue to make choices, both large and small, that influence our lives. We choose what work we will pursue, how we will treat others, and, of course, how we will care for our bodies. To be successful, we must start with a quality decision to submit ourselves to the Lord. We must choose to take up the role as the caretaker of God's temple, His dwelling place that He entrusted to us.

A quality decision is one that is well thought-out. We

want to make sure our decisions align with God and His Word, and that we understand the consequences of our choices. When we make a quality decision to do our part to care for our physical body, we are making a commitment to put our flesh under the authority of God's truth. While the untrained flesh may do some kicking and screaming at first, we know that the decision is right. So we keep moving forward to win the battle.

SO WHAT!

The messages we receive from the world are largely self-centered. We are constantly fed temptations to feed the flesh and its desires. We see advertisements for juicy hamburgers or mouth-watering desserts or sparkling beverages— all designed to feed the desires of the flesh, even though to consume them often wouldn't be good for our health. We are faced with an ongoing flow of temptations that feed the notion of "If I want it, I buy it" or "If I want it, I eat it." Consequently, we have people buried in debt and sick from lifestyle diseases.

As you gain understanding of the internal battle between your spirit and your flesh, I invite you to use this simple spiritual tool that will help you in just about every part of your life. I call it "So what!" It's part of putting the flesh in its place so we can stay on the course we chose.

The next time you sense a craving coming on, pause for a minute. Think about what is happening. Enter into your own "out-of-body experience" as you watch your flesh begging to be fed, and then say, "So what!"

So what if your flesh wants something that you know isn't good for you? Do you have to cater to the flesh and give in? No!

So what if you are being tempted by the enemy to give up your resolve? Do you need to crumble and let the wimp have his way? No!

So what if you have a craving? So what if you are tempted? So what if you have a twinge of wanting to give in, whether it's to food or another struggle in your life?

We seem to have given over so much of our internal power to our flesh, which is more aligned with the world than with the ways of God. Temptation isn't the problem; that's a natural part of life. It's what we do with temptation that can cause problems in our lives, just as we learn from God's Word:

> *No temptation has overtaken you except such as is*
> *common to man; but God is faithful, who will not*
> *allow you to be tempted beyond what you are able, but*
> *with the temptation will also make the way of escape,*
> *that you may be able to bear it.*
> 1 CORINTHIANS 10:13

> *Blessed is the man who endures temptation; for when*
> *he has been approved, he will receive the crown of life*
> *which the Lord has promised to those who love Him.*
> JAMES 1:12

While you are fasting you will very likely be tempted. Your flesh will send all kinds of signals to you, wanting foods or beverages that are not allowed on the Daniel Fast. But our Master Jesus practiced a proven remedy to counter these temptations. When He was in the wilderness and had been fasting from all food for forty days, His body wanted food. He was hungry—and maybe even vulnerable to temptation. Look at what happened:

> *Now when the tempter came to Him, he said, "If You are the Son of God, command that these stones become bread."*
>
> *But He answered and said, "It is written, 'Man shall not live by bread alone, but by every word that proceeds from the mouth of God.'"*
> MATTHEW 4:3-4

Jesus was tempted, but He did an internal "So what!" and then He answered the tempter with the antidote: "Man shall not live by bread alone, but by every word that proceeds from the mouth of God." Throughout the Scriptures we see this same remedy for temptation prescribed:

> *Watch and pray, lest you enter into temptation.*
> MATTHEW 26:41

> *When He came to the place, He said to them, "Pray that you may not enter into temptation."*
> LUKE 22:40

We do not live by bread alone. But what do we live by? Every word that proceeds from the mouth of God. We are called to watch and pray. To be aware of what is happening. To rely not on our own strength or willpower, but on the power of God working inside of us. We are told to invoke that power through our prayers.

Our faith walk toward the maturity in Christ we desire requires that we feed ourselves with good, nutritious food for the spirit, soul, and body. Each day we position ourselves for the abundant life we can have in Christ, and each day we need nourishment if we are to be strong and well-prepared for anything that could come against us.

CONSECRATION DURING YOUR FAST

We find the abundant life through submitting to God and His ways. Adhering to the choice to submit to God's authority can be challenging, especially when we are bombarded with temptations to go a different way. Here we see another powerful benefit of fasting. When we fast, we step into a different way of living for a period of time. We separate ourselves from our typical patterns and adopt distinct guidelines that we submit to and follow. We "consecrate ourselves," walking away from what is typical for us and into the holy fasting experience.

To consecrate means "to dedicate for a sacred purpose." Here we see God's instruction for the consecration of the Tabernacle in the Wilderness:

> *I will consecrate the tabernacle of meeting and the altar. I will also consecrate both Aaron and his sons to minister to Me as priests.*
> Exodus 29:44

God's instruction was that the Tabernacle, its furnishings, and the caretakers would be separated to be used of and for the Most High God. All was to be for holy purposes—godly purposes—His purposes.

But the separation doesn't end there in the wilderness. We, too, are called to be separate:

> *Therefore gird up the loins of your mind, be sober, and rest your hope fully upon the grace that is to be brought to you at the revelation of Jesus Christ; as obedient children, not conforming yourselves to the former lusts, as in your ignorance; but as He who called you is holy, you also be holy in all your conduct, because it is written, "Be holy, for I am holy."*
> 1 PETER 1:13-16

While we are always set apart by God because we have been redeemed by Him, we are "set apart" in another way when we are fasting. During your Daniel Fast, you will choose to walk according to the Spirit and away from the temptations of the flesh that show up around the foods you will restrict. And day by day, choice by choice, step by step, you will strengthen your faith muscles as you choose the ways of the fast. When your flesh starts to clamor for coffee, soda, candy, french fries, or whatever craving it decides to raise, you will say, "Sit down, flesh! You are out of order." You will take control of the flesh because you are choosing submission.

Now here is a hidden phenomenon that only those who

fast know about—and even then, only those who keep their spiritual life at the forefront of their fasting experience: You will begin to experience a greater division between the worldly-led part of you and the spirit-led part of you. Your spirit will take up more space in your thinking as your soul leans more and more toward God's ways. You will experience transformation. Look again at what God's Word teaches us:

> *I beseech you therefore, brethren, by the mercies of God,*
> *that you present your bodies a living sacrifice, holy,*
> *acceptable to God, which is your reasonable service. And*
> *do not be conformed to this world, but be transformed*
> *by the renewing of your mind, that you may prove what*
> *is that good and acceptable and perfect will of God.*
> ROMANS 12:1-2

Do you see it? Do you see how presenting your body is an act of submission and a choice to be consecrated? You are called to be holy, separated by God for His purposes as an act of service. Then as you follow this path of submission and consecration, you make choices that are aligned with God's ways. Your thinking is renewed, and transformation takes place. You continue to grow as you turn from the ways of the world and toward the ways of our Lord Jesus, again like Paul:

> *Not that I have already attained, or am already*
> *perfected; but I press on, that I may lay hold of that for*
> *which Christ Jesus has also laid hold of me. Brethren,*
> *I do not count myself to have apprehended; but one*

thing I do, forgetting those things which are behind
and reaching forward to those things which are ahead,
I press toward the goal for the prize of the upward call
of God in Christ Jesus.
PHILIPPIANS 3:12-14

God works in us! He performs masterful feats in our
souls. And it all starts when we make the quality decision
to follow Him and then choose His ways. We are renewed
in spirit, soul, and body—and we want to set our minds on
staying the course.

We take up our new way of Kingdom of God living. We
fully see ourselves as separated people, consecrated for the
Lord, and citizens of a different realm. The apostle Paul writes,

For our citizenship is in heaven, from which we also
eagerly wait for the Savior, the Lord Jesus Christ, who
will transform our lowly body that it may be conformed
to His glorious body, according to the working by which
He is able even to subdue all things to Himself.
PHILIPPIANS 3:20-21

Our life of faith is this continual and ongoing transformation process. We are God's chosen people. We are born
again. We are different. We are members of God's family.
Peter writes:

Coming to Him as to a living stone, rejected indeed
by men, but chosen by God and precious, you also,

as living stones, are being built up a spiritual house, a
holy priesthood, to offer up spiritual sacrifices acceptable
to God through Jesus Christ.

1 PETER 2:4-5

We are not of this world, but of the Kingdom of God, just as Jesus proclaimed when He prayed for His disciples and future believers:

They are not of the world, just as I am not of the world.
Sanctify them by Your truth. Your word is truth. As You
sent Me into the world, I also have sent them into the
world. And for their sakes I sanctify Myself, that they
also may be sanctified by the truth.

JOHN 17:16-19

We stay separated, on track, and strong in the Lord as we are sanctified by the truth found in God's living Word. The truth comes into us as we choose to open our hearts and minds to the Lord every single day. In this world, we are called to be lights. Our light stays bright as we continue to walk in the Spirit and submit our flesh to the ways of God.

WEIGHT LOSS SUCCESS TIP

If you experience food cravings, let the feeling serve as a signal that your body needs water, nutrition, or cleansing. Drink a tall glass of water. Eat a serving of fresh fruit or a few vegetables. You might want to munch on a small hand-ful of raw nuts. Once your body is well-nourished and well-hydrated, the cravings will disappear and you will be on your way toward your lifestyle of health.

CHAPTER 7

Ten Habits for Healthy Living

Creating Healthy Habits beyond the Fast

EXPERTS ON CHANGE say it takes about twenty-one days to develop a new habit. After that, it takes ninety days of using the new habit for it to actually become part of your lifestyle—something you do without thinking.

The twenty-one-day Daniel Fast can launch you into a healthier lifestyle. If you continue to use the new habits you develop during your fast, within about three months you will have a new way of being. You won't have to concentrate so much on the choices you make. Instead, you will have a new normal—a changed and healthy style of living.

Ever since I started teaching about the Daniel Fast, thousands of people have contacted me to ask about how they can continue on the healthy path they started traveling during their fast. Many wanted to fast forever, which is an oxymoron since fasting is always a temporary, highly focused, spiritual experience. But I knew what they were looking for. They wanted to stay within a system so they could continue to get stronger and healthier. They didn't want to go back to their old, unhealthy ways.

Their requests for help prompted me to start an online teaching forum that provides ongoing information, support, motivation, and encouragement. It's called Choose Life Now (Choose-Life-Now.com), and I praise God that He has used it to help so many women and men throughout the world. Members of Choose Life Now learn much of what I cover in this book. Over several months, they take continual steps to bring about healthy changes in their lives. Members start with submitting to God and learning more about how He wants them to care for their bodies.

Just as we can follow the example of people who are successful in managing money or raising children, we can look at the practices of people who live healthy lives. At Choose Life Now, members adopt a proven set of ten habits. They find that when these ten practices become permanent changes, they become healthier and shed pounds even though they aren't really even working at it.

Adopting these principles and making them your "way of being" comes with a guarantee that you will move into health and well-being.

TEN HABITS PRACTICED BY HEALTHY INDIVIDUALS

1. Eat small bites, chew them well, clear your mouth.
2. Drink lots of water.
3. Eat three meals a day.
4. Eat at least one meal each day at your dining table.

5. Quit the "Clean Plate Club."
6. Make a quality decision to eat for nutrition most of the time.
7. Let food be food.
8. Avoid the all-or-nothing mentality.
9. Get back on a healthy track the very next day after a splurge.
10. Don't deprive yourself of any food or food group.

1. Eat small bites, chew them well, clear your mouth. Take small bites (a size that fits comfortably on a fork and in your mouth); chew the food thoroughly until it's the consistency of applesauce; enjoy the flavors of your food while you're chewing; clear your mouth completely; and then take another small bite.

Most people are shocked at the significant difference this style of eating makes on the amount of food they eat and how much they enjoy their meals. Taking small bites and eating slowly allows your body to work as it was intended.

We eat primarily to provide nourishment for our bodies, and God planned our bodies with precision and function. When He designed the digestive system, He had it begin in our mouths. When we chew food, our teeth crush and grind it into smaller parts. As chewing continues, the food becomes softer and warmer. Glands in the mouth secrete saliva, and the enzymes in saliva begin to break down carbohydrates in the food. Then the food is swallowed for the next stage of digestion in the stomach.

Consider your tongue and its thousands of taste buds.

When you take a small bite, your taste receptors capture the flavors. Enjoying flavors is an essential reason for eating, along with nourishment. God created us to taste, and He created food to have flavors. However, a bigger bite doesn't increase the amount of flavor you taste. Instead, an oversized bite causes you to jostle the food in your mouth, and you oftentimes swallow it before it's completely chewed. Therefore, digestion is compromised, you've consumed extra calories, and your enjoyment is lessened.

God also created our bodies to give us signals so we know what actions to take. When the stomach has received enough food, it sends a signal to the brain to tell us to stop eating because it's had enough and is satisfied. This process takes about fifteen minutes. When you take oversized bites, eat fast, and don't chew your food well, your system's signaling functions go haywire. By the time your brain receives the signal that it's had enough to eat, you have already overconsumed.

Adopting the habit of taking small bites, chewing the food well to the consistency of applesauce while enjoying the flavors, swallowing to completely clear your mouth, and then taking another small bite allows your body to work in the way it was designed. You will enjoy your meals more. In addition, studies show that people who eat slowly consume 30 percent less food than those who rush their meals.

Try using this principle the next time you eat. First, be aware of your typical style of eating. Then, notice how you feel when you take small bites. Consider how much more you enjoy your food, and how much more quickly you sense the "enough food" sensation. Observe the length of time it takes you to eat, and then reflect on your overall experience. I think that you, like most people, will be very surprised.

2. Drink lots of water. Every part of your body depends on water for optimal operation. When it doesn't have adequate water, systems often break down. Developing the habit of drinking more water will bring dramatic improvements to your health. In addition, this practice will likely cause you to feel more full, so you eat less food and then drop more pounds.

Here is what I encourage people to do and try to practice myself: Plan to drink at least four tall glasses of water (sixteen ounces) each day. There are different opinions about this, but I prefer to drink water that is a little cooler than room temperature. The water goes down more easily and feels better in my stomach.

I drink one tall glass of water when I first get up in the morning, another fifteen to twenty minutes before lunch, and a third fifteen to twenty minutes before dinner. The fourth glass of water is sipped throughout the day. (I like to keep a glass or bottle of water with me at my desk, when I'm watching television, and in the car.)

When you are well hydrated, you will eat less food. When you drink a tall glass of water before meals, you will feel fuller. Plus, you are giving your body the water it needs so it won't send "thirsty" signals to your brain, which are often misread as hunger pangs.

Studies show that people who drink sixteen ounces

of water fifteen to twenty minutes before meals consume 30 percent less food than those who don't. That's good news!

3. Eat three meals a day. Your body needs nutrition, and it's designed to receive a consistent supply throughout the day. When you skip meals, your body reacts by storing more fat. In addition, when you skip meals, you are more likely to feel ravenously hungry and then overeat when you are around food. You are more likely to make poor food choices when you are responding to hunger rather than fulfilling a plan to nourish your body.

I encourage you to eat three healthy meals and two small snacks each day. It's a plan followed by many who are able to stay in good health.

4. Eat at least one meal each day at your dining table. We are an "on the go" culture. People often eat sitting at their desks, on the couch, in their cars, or even while standing or walking. The problem is, when dining is not your primary focus, it's easy to eat "unconsciously." In other words, your attention is focused on the book or report you are reading, the television show you are watching, the traffic you are driving in, or the conversation you are having, and you're not paying much attention to the food you are consuming.

Healthy people—women and men who are able to maintain healthy levels of weight—typically eat at least one meal every day at a dining table. Not only does this cut back on unconscious eating, but it also fosters relationships with family members. If you're married or have children at home, take a minute now to think about how you eat as a family. Do you dine together for your meals? Do you eat breakfast together? Do you share your dinner experience with one another and talk about what happened that day?

I get that families are busy these days. Eating all of our meals together may be impractical, especially with kids in school activities and sports. But coming together as a family (or as a couple if children are not in the home) is one of the best practices you can have for healthy family life and growth.

If you don't eat together as a family now, this might be the time to start. My adult children have thanked me numerous times for our practices of eating breakfast and dinner together at the dining table almost every day of each week. Whether you're married or single, live alone or in a full house, eating at least one meal a day at your dining table will help you to be more aware of what and how much you are eating.

5. Quit the "Clean Plate Club." People who maintain healthy weight stop eating as soon as their body sends them the signal that it's had enough to eat. Remember habit number one to take small bites, chew well, and clear your mouth? These two habits work really well together. Instead of feeling they need to eat every morsel of food on their plate, healthy people chose wellness over maintaining membership in the clean plate club.

Of course you can start by taking smaller portions to begin with, and then you won't feel like you are wasting food as often. But the key here is to make the choice that you will not overeat. When you first receive the signal that your body is satisfied and full, stop eating.

6. Make a quality decision to eat for nutrition most of the time. The primary purpose of food is to provide nourishment for your body. Pause. Take in this fact. Let it soak into your understanding.

So often, we think of food as being a delivery system for pleasure. While it's totally okay to enjoy our food, we want to keep the pleasure component in check—especially since an overabundance of desiring pleasure can quickly move into gluttony (ouch).

People who have a lifestyle of health eat primarily for nutrition most of the time. That means most of their meals are packed with vegetables, fruits, whole grains, legumes, small portions of animal proteins, and healthy oils. The meals can be delicious, but first they are nutritious. Then, on occasion, they waver from nutrition being first and go for the slice of decadent chocolate cake, the banana split, or even the potato chips with onion dip! The key is that eating like this is rare. It happens only occasionally, and so it doesn't cause a health problem.

You will find that when you follow this way of eating, just one bite of the decadent chocolate cake will satisfy your desire for something sweet, and you won't even want the whole piece. In fact, a recent study from Cornell University reported this finding:

> Eating smaller portions of commonly craved foods will satisfy a person just as well as a larger portion of the same food would.
>
> "This research supports the notion that eating

for pleasure—hedonic hunger—is driven more by the availability of foods instead of the food already eaten," said Brian Wansink, the John S. Dyson Professor of Marketing at Cornell's Dyson School of Applied Economics and Management and a co-author of the study, "Just a bite: Considerably smaller snack portions satisfy delayed hunger and craving."[1]

7. Let food be food. Healthy people don't eat because of stress, because they're bored, or because they just had a fight with their spouse. Healthy eaters let food be food. Not comfort. Not a pseudo-tranquilizer. Not a friend.

Overeaters often find themselves caught up in emotional eating, thinking that certain foods will make them feel better. The truth is, a bag of potato chips has never reached out and hugged you. A box of chocolates has never patted you on the back, and a carton of ice cream has never sung you a love song.

Let food be food. If you need emotional care, find it at the best Source: your Father who loves you more than you can ever measure. If you need to, call a friend who will let you vent, or find a healthy response that can give you the results you really want instead of more calories from fat, salt, and sugar. I find walking the best stress reliever for me. I can walk and pray or listen to uplifting music or an audio teaching.

Be your own private investigator. If you're eating food and you're not hungry and your body doesn't need nourishment, then take a minute to see what's going on inside of yourself. Be wise. Make a good choice.

8. Avoid the all-or-nothing mentality. Healthy eaters can take a few and leave the rest for later, whether it's potato chips, chocolates, or doughnuts. Do you remember the Alka-Seltzer commercial with the man sitting on the edge of his bed bemoaning, "I can't believe I ate the whole thing"? Clearly, he didn't avoid the all-or-nothing mentality.

One way to integrate this practice is never to eat out of boxes or bags of food. For example, if you plan to have some crackers, find out how many are in a serving. Then put that many on a small plate and eat them for a snack. If you pack lunches, place serving sizes in Ziploc bags and eat just one portion at a time. Think servings and not whole bags, whether it's chips, cookies, or candy.

9. Get back on a healthy track the very next day after a splurge. People who maintain a healthy weight may have the occasional celebration or feast, but then the next day they get right back to their normal healthy eating pattern. You can develop a lifestyle of health rather than one of overeating. Then on the rare occasion when you indulge, it's easy to snap right back into your normal ways.

Right now, you can make a quality decision—a resolution—to adopt this principle. Plan to return to your healthy way of eating if you splurge. Don't let your overconsumption or indulgence throw you off your path toward health.

10. Don't deprive yourself of any food or food group. This practice is linked to the one above. Healthy people don't totally deprive themselves of any specific food or food group, unless they are fasting or have medical issues to address. Deprivation only stirs desire and makes you want those chips or that chocolate cookie even more.

Obviously, this isn't talking about foods we should never eat because of our faith, such as marijuana-laced brownies or, in Daniel's time, food that had been offered to the Babylonian gods. That's a completely different issue. The deprivation I'm referring to is the kind dieters often use. They reason, "I can never eat ice cream again. Once I start, I can never stop." They cut out all ice cream, but the resolve usually doesn't last very long and they go back to overeating ice cream.

A better solution would be to practice these principles: Eat for health and stay nourished so your body isn't craving foods. Avoid the all-or-nothing way of thinking, and allow yourself a little of even unhealthy foods so you don't feel deprived.

WEIGHT LOSS SUCCESS TIP

Think about this: Two cups of fresh lettuce or spinach has fewer than fifteen calories. Add some sliced radishes and onions and a little salad dressing, and you have a large dinner salad for less than a hundred calories. Starting your meals with a low-calorie yet satisfying salad is a healthy and wise way to curb your appetite. You'll eat less and consume fewer calories for your meal, yet still have enough to eat. An added bonus is that salads provide the valuable fiber your body needs for good digestion, along with many micronutrients for your good health.

CHAPTER 8

The Shift

Submitting to God and Being Transformed

THE DANIEL FAST WILL LAUNCH YOUR JOURNEY toward a life-style of health. During the twenty-one days of fasting and following the plan, your body will undergo a measure of detoxing. You will be drinking more water and providing your internal systems the needed hydration for good health. It's very possible that you will become free of sugar addictions, if that is an issue, and you most likely will be shedding unwanted pounds.

You will have more energy as your body is able to function better. You will have a sense of well-being and vitality. Because your blood sugar levels are stable, your sleep will probably be of better quality, and your moods will be more steady and grounded. Best of all, you will be motivated and encouraged by your successful experience.

As you contemplate the teachings in this book about who you are in Christ—that you are the temple of God's Holy

Spirit and a valuable member of God's family—you will experience a change in your attitudes about food and your health. When you couple these changes with the new habits for healthy living we looked at in the last chapter, you will be well on your way to a lifestyle of health and well-being.

If you're reading these words before you start your fast, these transitions may seem impossible. And they will be if you try to do this from your own strength rather than by incorporating your faith and God's power. But we know that God Himself is working within us, making us who we were created to be. Philippians 1:6 reminds us, "He who has begun a good work in you will complete it until the day of Jesus Christ." We are not doing this on our own. With God's help, we will be transformed. We will change.

THE SHIFT IS COMING

Here is what you can look forward to if you stay the course: You will have a day when you walk down the aisle at the grocery store and you aren't even tempted by the sugary, fatty, or salty foods that used to be your downfall. You'll realize that food no longer has a hold on you, and that it's no longer on the pedestal it once was on. You will experience a shift, and at first, it might even come as a surprise to you.

Years ago when I went to a movie theater, my usual practice would be to get a large soda and a jumbo tub of buttered popcorn—you know, the one with free refills! I would share the popcorn with whoever I was with for the film. We could easily down one, if not two, tubs of movie popcorn and even have some to take home.

Then I learned about how bad movie theater popcorn is for my body, plus my outlook changed about how important it is for me to care for my health. The next time I walked into the theater I didn't even want the popcorn and soda. The appeal was gone. My "before" was, "Oh, I love the popcorn they make at that movie theater." My "after" was, "No thanks. I'm not interested." It wasn't, "I really want the popcorn, but I know it's not good for me. I will stay strong and not get it." No, I really didn't even want it. I had no desire. The cravings were nonexistent.

That's the shift. I'm confident that you will have similar experiences. You will find that food no longer has the control over you it once had. Foods that you once craved and overate won't tempt you anymore, and some won't even be appetizing.

SUDDENLY AFTER A WHILE

When can you expect this kind of deeply rooted change? I can only say, "Sooner and later." You will notice some changes soon, while others will unfold over time.

When I was a teenager—oh, this is hard to imagine— I craved Hostess CupCakes. I even enjoyed the occasional Twinkie. When I was in high school, I would sometimes eat only Hostess CupCakes and a carton of milk for lunch! My body is cringing now as I remember those days.

Today, I can no more imagine eating either of those foods than eating sand. It's been decades since I wanted them. Clearly, my tastes have changed. Over time I adopted other levels of healthy eating, and as a young adult my tastes in food changed toward healthier choices. I became a fan of brown rice long before it was popular, and highly processed foods weren't very appetizing to me.

However, it was when I started using the Daniel Fast as my method of fasting that I changed the most. Obviously, on the fast I followed a completely plant-based eating plan. When the fast was over, I just continued eating a lot of the same recipes I had prepared during the fast. I lost my appetite for cow's milk, which is often packed with antibiotics, hormones, and genetically modified substances, and now I use only unsweetened soy or almond milk. I rarely drink it, but instead use it in recipes or on cereal. These days, I eat much less meat and many more vegan dishes. I keep nuts in my cupboards as a staple and usually turn to them first when I want a snack. These changes that started with the Daniel Fast took a few years to carry over into my everyday life and eventually became my way of living. The changes were natural and didn't require a lot of strong willpower. Instead, they were bit-by-bit changes.

Then I started learning more about health and the food industry. I learned that most non-organic animal products are from stock that has been fed lots of chemicals or has received growth hormones and antibiotics. Those drugs are in their meat, milk, cheese, and whatever foods end up in our grocery stores. I made a health-based decision to buy only organically raised animal proteins.

When I learned more about the vital role water plays in the body, I started drinking more water each day. When I'm not fasting, I also drink a lot of green tea, which has many health benefits. I enjoy the flavor of the hot drink, especially on cold winter days. Again, when I'm not fasting, I enjoy a cup of steaming hot coffee in the morning. I admit, giving up coffee during the Daniel Fast is the most challenging part of the food restrictions for me. In part that's because I miss the flavor, but mostly I miss it because it is part of my daily routine of getting up before dawn, making coffee, and then sipping it while I greet the Lord and spend one-on-One time with Him. I keep the routine when I fast, but instead of hot coffee, I drink hot water, sometimes with a slice of lemon.

I used to drink half-and-half cream in my coffee. In fact, I was kind of a snob about it. I had to have organic half-and-half—not milk, not creamer. Only the real stuff! If I was somewhere that didn't have it, I would just drink the coffee black. Eventually I realized the extra calories from the half-and-half were adding to my diet, and I decided to cut it out. That was a few years ago. I still enjoy my morning cup of coffee, but it's black all the time.

As I learned more about the huge health advantages of eating more fruits and vegetables, I made a point to eat more salads and more steamed vegetables on a daily basis. I don't always make it, but I try to have at least one large salad each day and one large helping of slightly steamed vegetables.

All these changes toward improved health came about slowly. They were natural changes that were motivated both from knowledge and from my desire to be healthy. I'm now at a place where I eat in a very healthy way most of the time. Rarely do I eat desserts or sugary foods. I will have the occasional piece of dark chocolate, which not only can satisfy a now much tamer sweet tooth, but is actually loaded with nutrients and is one of the best sources for antioxidants. I still like to bake, and I'll make cookies or bread for a special occasion. I'll even eat some potato chips a few times a year. However, now I truly can take them or leave them. They don't have a hold on me!

This shift is due in part to my changed eating habits leading to changed food preferences. But it's also because I am nourishing my body better than ever, and a nourished body is a satisfied body. The systems are all working in harmony, so I don't have the sugar spikes or the signs of dehydration that are often mistaken for hunger pangs.

I can still make some improvements for my health. As our bodies age, we need to be more diligent about exercise, stretching, and stamina. I can still eat more fresh vegetables and drink more water. But over the years, I have been transformed. No matter what your health struggles and eating habits have been, I'm confident that you can see positive change. If you take what you've learned during this fast and adopt healthy habits going forward, you will see transformation in your life too.

INTEGRATION OF THE SPIRIT, SOUL, AND BODY

Jesus teaches us to "seek first the kingdom of God and His righteousness," or His right way of doing things (see Matthew 6:33). We always want to begin everything with God and His ways. When we get into the Scriptures and learn what the Lord has to say about who we are and how we should care for our bodies, there should be only one love-loaded response to our Lord: "Yes, Sir." He is our number one reason for making changes to be better aligned with what He wants for us. He wants us to be healthy. He wants us to take good care of our bodies. He wants us to be a shining example of His family.

Our response to the Daniel Fast encompasses all aspects—the spirit, soul, and body. First, we decide to enter into this fasting experience and present our bodies as a living sacrifice unto the Lord because we are God's. He bought us with a price and we are His. He is our reason to drop unwanted pounds and turn toward health and well-being. Our foundation for change is to be led by the Spirit and have our own spirits respond in humility and love.

We make choices and point our attention toward learning about health with our minds, which are the soul part of us. It is our soul that submits to God. It is with our soul that we open our minds to God's truth and also to learning about how He created us and how to best take care of our bodies. When God made us, He put our souls in the position of governance over our lives. We are in charge of making choices, and we decide if we will submit to God or do things our own way. He sets before us life and death, blessing and cursing—and then He tells us to choose life. A soul submitted to the Lord makes that choice.

Finally, our body is the place where we are housed along with God. He is in us. And when we accept Jesus and make Him the Lord of our lives, we transfer ownership of our bodies to Him. He bought us with the price of His blood.

Our spirit, soul, and body are aligned with God when

we lovingly submit to Him and make the quality decision to follow His ways. That is when we are fully integrated and one with the Father and the Son. Submission fuels the transformation, which allows the shift to happen. Even if it doesn't seem attainable to you now, trust in the power of God to change you.

WEIGHT LOSS SUCCESS TIP

As you plan your meals and snacks, make sure each menu includes protein. Whole grains, green leafy vegetables, nuts, and seeds are all good sources. Protein not only supplies your body with the nutrients needed to regenerate cells and provide energy, but it also makes you feel full and satisfied over several hours. Eating healthy proteins complemented with fruits and vegetables will avoid sugar highs and lows and carry you to your next meal.

CHAPTER 9

Keeping It Going

Staying on the Path of Lasting Change

I CAN'T COUNT THE NUMBER of messages I've received from disappointed women and men who felt so great while they were on the Daniel Fast and then tried to keep their new habits going after the fast was over. Unfortunately, they fell back into old patterns of unhealthy consumption and over-eating. They write asking when there will be another group Daniel Fast because they want to get back on the road that was leading them to health.

Here is the problem with just repeating the same actions: It didn't work the first time. What will these people do differently the next time to lead them to the success they want?

I believe the key to making lasting change to fundamental parts of our lives, including eating, is first to change on the inside. That's why I am writing this book.

I know the power of the Daniel Fast and the almost-too-good-to-be-true effects it can have on people's health. I've seen it in my own life and in the lives of tens of thousands of others. With that said, I am totally against turning the Daniel Fast into a diet plan or entering into the sacred discipline of fasting with food as the focus. That approach will only change people externally and temporarily, and they will miss the priceless treasure and internal change available to anyone who embarks on a Spirit-driven fast.

I hope that in this book I have been able to present a Christ-centered platform where people who know they need to change their eating habits can find help that leads to lasting solutions. My goal is to guide you into a meaningful fasting experience that focuses on who you are in Christ and the opportunities and responsibilities you have as a child of God to pursue health.

Jesus revealed to anyone who would listen with spiritual ears that "the kingdom of God is within you" (Luke 17:21). Change on the outside comes when we first change the inside—how we think and what we believe to be true. When we invest the time to meditate on God's truths, they can become deeply rooted in our hearts. From there, change erupts and will soon and very soon turn into a renewed way of living.

Solomon wrote about God's wisdom being life and health to those who heed it:

My son, give attention to my words;
Incline your ear to my sayings.
Do not let them depart from your eyes;
Keep them in the midst of your heart;
For they are life to those who find them,

And health to all their flesh.
Keep your heart with all diligence,
For out of it spring the issues of life.

PROVERBS 4:20-23

God's ways are the best path for life. When we keep
His truth at the forefront of our minds, we will experience
renewal—spirit, soul, and body. And it can be lasting! Later
in the same passage, Solomon makes an essential point about
how to stay the course, once you're on it:

Put away from you a deceitful mouth,
And put perverse lips far from you.
Let your eyes look straight ahead,
And your eyelids look right before you.
Ponder the path of your feet,
And let all your ways be established.
Do not turn to the right or the left;
Remove your foot from evil.

PROVERBS 4:24-27

That's a powerful visual image of focus: We put aside our
temptations and distractions, and we keep our eyes focused
on the goal. Paul gave the Philippians similar advice when
he taught them how to stay on course with their new way
of living:

Beloved, I do not consider that I have made it my own;
but this one thing I do: forgetting what lies behind and

straining forward to what lies ahead, I press on toward the goal for the prize of the heavenly call of God in Christ Jesus. Let those of us then who are mature be of the same mind; and if you think differently about anything, this too God will reveal to you. Only let us hold fast to what we have attained.

Philippians 3:13-16, NRSV

If you want to have a healthy lifestyle, you first need to make sure that the biblical truths shared here are deeply rooted in your soul. That change will determine your choices. And as you keep walking straight forward, not turning to the right or to the left, you will reach the destination you desire—which is the one your Creator wants for you also.

Remember these words from Ecclesiastes: "Though one may be overpowered by another, two can withstand him. And a threefold cord is not quickly broken" (Ecclesiastes 4:12). The three "strands" of the cord in this case are first of all God, then sound and proven principles, and finally you and your resolve to stay the course. If you find your resolve crumbling, it's likely because you're not utilizing all three cords. To get back on track, conduct a self-assessment. Are you relying solely on yourself and forgetting that God is at work? Have you neglected some of the principles and habits that will help you through? Has your resolve slipped? Discover what you are missing, and then make the adjustments. The key is to get back on the road to health. Get back on the path that will lead you to the destination you want to reach.

TRANSITIONING OFF THE DANIEL FAST

During your Daniel Fast, you will eat very healthy foods and drink gallons of refreshing, cleansing water. But what happens when the fast is done? How can you transition back to unrestricted eating without losing the health you have gained in the past weeks?

First, think about what foods you will eat. Some of the foods not allowed on the fast you can keep off your list forever! That's just a good plan for your health and well-being. But other foods not allowed on the fast are good for your health, and you may enjoy them. Including those back into your eating plan is fine. The key is to exercise the principle to "Eat for good nutrition most of the time."

I encourage people to use the Daniel Fast eating plan as their core diet, and then add small portions of lean animal proteins and low-fat dairy into their menus. Continue to drink at least four tall glasses of water each day. If you want to drink coffee, tea, and other beverages, keep your health in mind and remember that you are the caretaker of the temple of the Holy Spirit, and you want to do a good job.

Plan your meals for nourishment and then for pleasure. Develop a set of five or six core menus with recipes that use beneficial ingredients. Get really good at preparing the recipes, perfecting them to your individual liking and the tastes of your family. You'll find many ideas in the recipe section of this book. Stock up on good quality foods so they are available when you need to prepare a meal or when you want a snack. Take advantage of sales on frozen and canned products that provide nutritious ingredients, and minimize the amount of junk food in your cupboards.

Develop a plan for healthy snacking and keep the ingredients on hand in your pantry. Nuts, popcorn, hummus, vegetables, and fruits are all good options for healthy snacking, and soon these will be your preferred choices.

During times of celebration and feasting, it's appropriate and even good to "color outside of the lines" for your menus. Holidays often include many rich and sweet foods. Birthdays have cakes. Big sporting events have chips and sodas. You will remain within the boundaries of healthy living if you partake in the celebrations and eat some of the foods offered, but then the next day return to your healthy eating patterns. No harm, no foul. All is well.

The Bread of Life

Along with developing a healthy eating plan for your physical body once you're finished with the fast, you will also want to stay on course by providing ample food for your spirit. Keeping your resolve strong will depend on remaining firmly rooted in the ways of the Lord.

Keep a list of verses in your Bible that you can refer to frequently for meditation, praise, and prayer. These verses can serve as signposts to keep you on track and moving in the direction you want to travel. Also, if at some point during your day you sense you are ready to move off your desired path, pause and pray. Center yourself on the truth in your heart. Order your flesh to sit down and behave, and make a healthy choice. Drink some water. Munch on some nuts or a piece of fruit. Most of the time you will find that the temptation will pass within twenty minutes.

If you still have the craving, then apply healthy principle number 8: "Avoid the all-or-nothing mentality." Take a small bite of the desired food, enjoy the flavors, and be satisfied.

If the cravings persist, then this could be a warning sign that you are headed in the wrong direction. Don't merely pause at this point. Instead, take a careful look at the direction you are heading, make the appropriate adjustments, and see it through.

Feed Your Soul

In chapter 3 we learned the power of knowledge and understanding. As you continue on your journey toward a lifestyle of health, you will want to feed your mind with good information about health, nutrition, and good living. Make the practice of informing yourself about health part of your lifestyle.

This doesn't need to be hard or too time consuming. Some excellent television programs provide useful information about nutrition and healthy living, and you can find many good books at your local or online bookstore or at your local library. Over the last several years, filmmakers have produced some outstanding documentaries about health, the food industry, and nutrition. My personal favorites are magazines that I subscribe to so I can keep a constant flow of current and useful information coming into my home to feed my mind.

Please don't overlook the power of consistently feeding

your whole being with healthy food for your spirit, soul, and body. Not only will this provide the health you want, but it will also build up defenses and protect you from outside invaders that can do you harm. It puts you on the path to good health.

STAYING ON THE PATH

Do you remember back in chapter 2 when I talked about walking the five-hundred-mile Camino de Santiago across northern Spain? While I shared this journey with a friend of mine, she and I rarely walked together since we had different paces. Plus, we both were on the journey to spend copious amounts of one-on-One time with God.

When you walk the Camino, you usually carry a guide-book, but you don't follow a map to see when to turn right, go straight, or turn left. Instead, you're directed by yellow arrows painted on the sides of buildings, small signs, the road, stones, or wherever is necessary so the pilgrims can stay on the right path and keep moving toward Santiago.

On one particular day, I was walking alone as I usually did. The yellow arrows pointed me to walk on the sidewalks through a small town. Then more yellow arrows pointed me to a path veering away from the village and off into the countryside.

I had walked what would be about two city blocks away from the town when I heard a horn honking. I turned around to see where the sound was coming from and saw a small truck at the head of the path I was walking on. I thought whoever was in the truck was honking to alert someone in one of the nearby apartments that he was there to pick them up, so I turned and kept walking.

But then the honking didn't stop. I turned around again to look, and this time I saw a man standing outside of his truck, still honking the horn, but now waving his arms at me.

This was odd. Why in the world would he be summoning me?

I wasn't sure, but I could see that he really wanted my attention. I turned around and walked back down the pathway to his truck so I could see what he wanted.

My Spanish isn't the greatest, and I quickly learned that his English was nonexistent. But thankfully we could communicate through our facial expressions and hand motions. He pointed in the direction where I had been walking and said, "No, no." Then he proceeded to show me a small yellow arrow off to the right. It pointed to a hairpin turn that led to a small tunnel under the road. I had missed the yellow arrow, and the very kind man used his horn to warn me that I was walking in the wrong direction—which, by the way, could have taken me miles and miles away from the Camino route!

My heart filled with thanksgiving for this dear man who took the time to warn me of my mistake. Even now I am touched as I remember his act of kindness toward me. Our smiles to each other exchanged the words we could not express, and then we both went our separate ways.

If I had not heeded the warnings, I would have walked in the opposite direction of where I really wanted to go. Thankfully, this kind man with his persistence got my attention and pointed me in the right direction.

I hope to be serving you in that same manner. I hope you are reading these words and hearing deep in your heart the call to health . . . and seeing that if you want to get there, you need to change the direction you are walking. Maybe you're like me and need to make a 180-degree turnaround and start walking in the opposite direction. Or perhaps you're just a little off course, but you know that even a few degrees can keep you from reaching the destination of your dreams.

You can start right away and get on the path. As we see in Proverbs, "Ponder the path of your feet, and let all your ways be established. Do not turn to the right or the left; remove your foot from evil" (Proverbs 4:26-27). Stay on the course with joy in your heart and assurance in each step you take that you will reach the place you are going, one step at a time.

WEIGHT LOSS SUCCESS TIP

Planning and simplicity are a dynamic duo on your journey toward a lifestyle of health. So often when we're tired and hungry, we reach for quick and easy food solutions—but those are frequently packed with sugar, fat, salt, and processed ingredients. However, if you plan ahead and have simple, easy-to-make meals on hand, you are more likely to stay on your desired path and eat nutritious foods that are good for you.

PART TWO

Daniel Fast Recipes
for Weight Loss

The LORD God planted a garden eastward in Eden, and there He put the man whom He had formed. And out of the ground the LORD God made every tree grow that is pleasant to the sight and good for food.

GENESIS 2:8-9

WHEN GOD CREATED EDEN, the perfect place for human beings to live and grow, He provided good food to nourish Adam and Eve's bodies. He knew exactly what their beautiful and intricately designed systems would need to stay in perfect health. Plus, He provided for their sensory pleasure and enjoyment. Everything in the Garden was lovely to look at and released a delightful fragrance.

While we're no longer in the Garden of Eden, we can still enjoy the beautiful and healthy foods God created. As you think about your wonderfully designed body, which God has entrusted to your care, consider what you will allow to enter it. Make a quality decision to nourish your body with the good and perfect foods that our Lord created just for us. As you practice this way of eating as a lifestyle, you will be giving His temple just what it needs for health and vitality.

PLANNING AND PREPARATION

You want to set yourself up for success as you get ready for your fast. A key element of a positive outcome is to plan your meals. I strongly encourage you to keep your meals simple and easy to prepare. Here are ten tips to help you succeed with meal planning and preparation:

1. Develop five or six dinner meals that you can focus on as you begin your fast. Select menus that you know you and your family will like and that fit with your lifestyle, even as you fast. Plan to use leftovers or partial portions for your lunch menus. You can rotate these menus during your entire fasting period to keep meal preparation simple.

2. Choose three breakfast meals that you will use as you begin the fast, plus three snacks that you can have handy at home, in your car, and at work or school.

3. Plan a complete week of menus, including breakfast, lunch, dinner, and snacks. You can go to Daniel-Fast.com/mealplanner for a handy worksheet that has everything on one page.

4. Make a shopping list of all the ingredients you need for your menus and shop for a full week of meals in one outing.

5. When you return from your shopping trip, wash, prepare, and store all your salad ingredients so they are ready throughout the week. You will be amazed at how quickly you can make a salad when all the ingredients are already sliced and ready to go.

6. Consider having a "cooking day" where you prepare several meals that you can then store or freeze to use in the week. This is the cook-once-eat-several-times approach and will save you hours of time during the week.

7. Use your cooking day as a time to feed your soul. Listen to worship music or Bible teachings. Pray or memorize Scripture. Turn what can be a task-time into a positive and uplifting experience.

8. Make your own "snack bags" by purchasing small snack-sized Ziploc plastic bags and then filling them with one serving of a snack, such as ¼ cup raw or seasoned nuts, sliced veggies, or sliced fruit.

9. Make sure you have Daniel Fast food available so you can stay within the guidelines at those moments when you are short of time or experiencing cravings. If you plan for those challenging times, you will be prepared when they occur.

10. Engage the family in meal planning and preparation. This can be especially helpful for youngsters. Their involvement in preparing more vegetables and fruits for their meals can also increase their desire to consume them.

THE DANIEL FAST FOOD LIST

The Daniel Fast is a totally plant-based, whole food eating plan, and the only beverage is water. All foods are free of sweeteners, chemicals, and artificial colorings and flavorings. No processed foods are allowed, meaning those whole foods that have been altered by the food manufacturers, such as white flour or white rice where the original grain has been separated and the germ and hull removed, leaving only the starchy portion of the grain.

Unsweetened juice may be used in recipes; however, keep in mind that the only beverage on the Daniel Fast is water.

Foods to Include in Your Diet during the Daniel Fast

All fruits. These can be fresh, frozen, dried, juiced, or canned. Fruits include but are not limited to apples, apricots, bananas, blackberries, blueberries, boysenberries, cantaloupe, cherries, cranberries, figs, grapefruit, grapes, guava, honeydew melon, kiwi, lemons, limes, mangoes, nectarines, oranges, papayas, peaches, pears, pineapples, plums, prunes, raisins, raspberries, strawberries, tangelos, tangerines, and watermelon.

All vegetables. These can be fresh, frozen, dried, juiced, or canned. Vegetables include but are not limited to artichokes, asparagus, beets, broccoli, Brussels sprouts, cabbage, carrots, cauliflower, celery, chili peppers, collard greens, corn, cucumbers, eggplant, garlic, gingerroot, kale, leeks, lettuce, mushrooms, mustard greens, okra, onions, parsley, potatoes, radishes, rutabagas, scallions, spinach, sprouts, squashes, sweet potatoes, tomatoes, turnips, watercress, yams, and zucchini. Veggie burgers are also an option if you are not allergic to soy.

All whole grains, including but not limited to whole wheat, brown rice, millet, quinoa, oats, barley, grits, whole wheat pasta, whole wheat tortillas, rice cakes, and popcorn.

All nuts and seeds, including but not limited to sunflower seeds, cashews, peanuts, and sesame seeds. Also nut butters, including peanut butter.

All legumes. These can be canned or dried. Legumes include but are not limited to dried beans, pinto beans, split peas, lentils, black-eyed peas, kidney beans, black beans, cannellini beans, white beans.

All quality oils, including but not limited to olive, canola, grape-seed, peanut, and sesame.

Beverages: spring water, distilled water, or other pure waters.

Other: tofu, soy products, vinegar, seasonings, salt, herbs, and spices.

Foods to Avoid on the Daniel Fast

All meat and animal products, including but not limited to beef, lamb, pork, poultry, fish, and eggs.

All dairy products, including but not limited to milk, cheese, cream, and butter.

All sweeteners, including but not limited to sugar, raw sugar, honey, syrups, molasses, date honey, and cane juice.

All leavened bread, including but not limited to Ezekiel Bread (most of which contains yeast and honey), pretzels, pita bread, and other baked goods made with leavening agents.

All refined and processed food products, including but not limited to artificial flavorings, food additives, chemicals, white rice, white flour, and foods that contain artificial preservatives.

All deep fried foods, including but not limited to potato chips, French fries, and corn chips.

All solid fats, including shortening, butter, margarine, lard, and foods high in fat.

All nonwater beverages, including but not limited to coffee, tea, herbal teas, carbonated beverages, energy drinks, and alcohol.

Remember, *read the labels* and study the list of ingredients included in any packaged food to ensure that the contents comply with the Daniel Fast guidelines.

RECIPES

In the next pages you will find a variety of recipes that you can use for your twenty-one-day Daniel Fast. As you prepare your meals, think about how you are giving your body the nourishment it needs for good health. Thank God for creating colorful and appetizing ingredients that you can mix into flavorful recipes. From breakfasts to lunches, snacks, and main dishes, you'll gain ideas for how to prepare meals that will keep you satisfied and nourished.

As I've said before, the Daniel Fast is not a diet plan, and there's no need to count calories. Food allowed on the fast is healthy food, and so as we eat, we can think about choosing well rather than about limiting ourselves. However, people who are trying to lose weight sometimes want to know which foods they should eat in moderation and which they can eat freely. With that in mind, we've highlighted those recipes that are particularly low in calories with this special icon: ✓ .

Breakfasts

Basic Scrambled Tofu

INGREDIENTS
- ½ yellow onion, diced
- ½ green bell pepper, seeded and diced
- 1 14-ounce block firm tofu, drained
- 2 tablespoons olive oil
- 1 teaspoon garlic powder
- 1 teaspoon onion powder
- 1 tablespoon unsweetened soy sauce
- ½ teaspoon turmeric (optional)
- Salt and freshly ground black pepper to taste

1. Using a sharp knife, cut the tofu into one-inch cubes and then gently crumble with clean hands or a fork.

2. Heat the oil in a medium skillet over medium-high heat. Add the onion, pepper, and crumbled tofu; sauté for 3–5 minutes while stirring often. Add the garlic powder, onion powder, soy sauce, and turmeric; reduce the heat to medium and cook 5–7 more minutes, stirring frequently. Add additional oil if needed. Season to taste.

3. Serve with fresh fruit or wrapped in a tortilla for a breakfast wrap.

Makes 2 servings

Black Bean Breakfast Bowl

INGREDIENTS
- 2 tablespoons olive oil
- 1 14-ounce block firm tofu, drained and crumbled
- 1 teaspoon garlic powder
- 1 teaspoon onion powder
- 1 can (15 ounces) black beans, drained and rinsed
- 1 avocado, peeled and sliced

- ¼ cup salsa
- Salt and freshly ground black pepper to taste

1. Heat the olive oil in a small skillet over medium heat. Add the crumbled tofu and gently stir in the onion powder and garlic powder. Heat for 3–5 minutes.

2. Heat the black beans in the microwave by placing them in a microwave-safe bowl and heating on high for 1–2 minutes.

3. Divide the warmed black beans into two individual serving bowls.

4. Top each bowl with scrambled tofu, avocado, and salsa. Season with salt and black pepper.

Makes 2 servings

Breakfast Tofu and Veggie Scramble

INGREDIENTS
- 1 tablespoon olive oil
- ½ cup finely chopped yellow onion
- ½ cup chopped red bell pepper
- ½ cup frozen peas
- ½ cup frozen corn
- 1 teaspoon ground cumin
- 12 ounces firm tofu, cubed and then crumbled
- Salt and freshly ground pepper to taste

1. Heat the oil in a large skillet over medium-high heat. Add the onion and sauté until it softens and becomes translucent.

2. Stir in the red bell pepper, peas, corn, and cumin; cook for 2–3 minutes. Reduce the heat to low and add the tofu. Gently toss to blend with the vegetables.

3. Continue to cook until the tofu is warm; season with salt and pepper to taste.

4. Serve with slices of fresh fruit for a nutritious meal.

Makes 2 servings

Homemade Muesli Cereal

INGREDIENTS
- 5 cups rolled oats (1 pound)
- 2 teaspoons ground cinnamon
- ½ cup walnuts, roughly broken
- ¼ cup sliced almonds
- ½ cup raw sunflower seeds
- ½ cup toasted wheat germ
- ½ cup dried apricots, coarsely chopped
- ½ cup golden raisins
- ½ cup raisins
- ½ cup dried apples, coarsely chopped

1. Heat oven to 375 degrees.

2. Mix the oats with the cinnamon and then spread the mixture on a baking sheet. Place in preheated oven and toast for 15 minutes.

3. Toast the walnuts for about 10 minutes; toast the almonds for about 4 minutes.

4. When all ingredients are cool, toss together the toasted nuts with oats. Then add the sunflower seeds, wheat germ, and dried fruit.

5. Serve with hot or cold unsweetened plant-based milk and fresh berries.

Makes about 8 cups. Each serving is about ¼ cup.

Stored in an airtight jar, the muesli will keep for several weeks.

Hot Oatmeal

Oatmeal comes in three varieties: quick-cooking oats, rolled oats, and steel-cut oats. The variety you choose depends on your personal preference and the time you have to prepare your meal. Be sure to read the list of ingredients on the packages of oats to make sure no sweeteners or chemicals have been added.

Quick-Cooking Oats

INGREDIENTS
- ½ cup oats
- 1 cup water or unsweetened plant-based milk
- Pinch of salt

1. Combine ingredients in a microwavable bowl.

2. Cook in the microwave for 1½–2 minutes on high.

3. Stir in unsweetened plant-based milk and serve with fresh or dried fruit.

Makes 1 serving

Old-Fashioned Rolled Oats

INGREDIENTS
- 1 cup water or unsweetened plant-based milk
- Pinch of salt
- ½ cup old-fashioned rolled oats

1. Pour the water or milk into a small saucepan. Add the salt and slowly bring to a boil over medium-high heat.

2. Stir in the oats and reduce the heat to medium. Cook for 5 minutes, stirring occasionally. Cover, remove from heat, and let stand for 2–3 minutes.

3. Serve with fresh or dried fruit.

Makes 1 serving

Steel-Cut Oats

Since these oats are not rolled, they take longer to cook, but the texture is delightful.

INGREDIENTS
- 1 cup steel-cut oats
- 4½ cups water
- 1 cup mixed dried fruit
- ½ cup chopped mixed nuts and seeds

1. Place all ingredients in a slow cooker; gently stir to blend.

2. Set the heat to low and cook for 8–9 hours.

3. Serve with warmed unsweetened plant-based milk.

Makes 4 servings

Steel-Cut Oats in a Jar

This is a handy "make ahead" meal that you can prepare while you are cooking other meals and then use in the mornings. Be creative with your toppings and enjoy these nutrition-packed jars of goodness.

INGREDIENTS
- 1⅔ cups steel-cut oats
- 4 cups water
- ¼ teaspoon salt

Additional ingredients
- Unsweetened plant-based milk
- Cinnamon, nutmeg, or other spices
- Raisins, apricots, apples, or other dried fruit
- Nuts and seeds

Note: You will need 5 pint-sized wide-mouthed canning jars with lids.

1. Place the oats, water, and salt in a medium-sized saucepan and bring to a boil over medium-high heat. Reduce the heat and simmer for about 3 minutes, stirring a few times to prevent sticking. Turn off the heat.

2. Using a ladle, evenly distribute the oats-and-water mixture into the jars. Cover the jars tightly with their caps and rings, and then leave on the counter overnight.

3. The next morning the oats will be soft and ready to eat. You can add spices, nuts, and dried fruit to each of the jars according to your taste. Reseal the lids and then place all the jars in the refrigerator.

4. When you're ready to eat a jar of oatmeal, remove the lid and ring and microwave right in the jar for 2–3 minutes, or until it is hot enough for your liking. Add the unsweetened plant-based milk and enjoy!

5. The next day, repeat step 4 with another jar, and you have a nutritious, delicious breakfast in minutes. Use within 4 days.

Makes 5 servings

Rice Cakes with Toppings

I realize this isn't the typical recipe you find in a cookbook. But in keeping with the "simple is better" mode of operation when it comes to preparing healthy meals for your Daniel Fast and beyond, I want to add this simple breakfast or snack idea. I keep most of these ingredients in my cupboards so they are available when I need them.

INGREDIENTS
- 1 whole-grain rice cake
- Your choice of spread and topping

1. Spread the rice cake with an ingredient of your choice (see the idea list below).

2. Add one or more toppings (see ideas below).

Spreads:

• Peanut butter (or other nut butters you may like)

• Hummus

• Bean Dip

• Guacamole

Ideas for toppings:

- Apple, thinly sliced
- Avocado, thinly sliced
- Chopped nuts
- Dried fruit
- Raisins
- Salsa
- Sliced bananas

Makes 1 serving

Smoothies

Banana and Cashew Cream Smoothie

INGREDIENTS
- 1 cup boiling water
- 1 cup raw cashews
- 1 banana
- 1 cup ice
- 1 teaspoon pure vanilla extract

1. Place cashews in a blender. Pour the boiling water over them and cover. Let stand until softened, about 15 minutes.

2. Puree in the blender on high speed until smooth, about 3 minutes.

3. Add the banana and puree again. Add ice and vanilla extract; blend until smooth. If necessary, add a bit of water to reach desired consistency.

Makes 2 servings

Berry-Banana Breakfast Smoothie

INGREDIENTS
- 2 cups unsweetened almond milk
- ¼ cup unsweetened coconut milk
- 1 cup frozen blueberries
- 1 cup frozen peaches, mango, or pineapple (or a mix)
- 1 ripe banana
- ½ cup fresh spinach
- 2 tablespoons chia seeds
- 1 tablespoon flax seeds
- 1 teaspoon vanilla extract (optional)

1. Combine all ingredients in a blender. Puree until smooth, about 1 minute. The smoothie should be thick, so if needed, add more frozen fruit until the desired consistency is reached.

2. Serve immediately.

Makes 2 servings

Easy Berry-Nut Breakfast Smoothie

INGREDIENTS
- ½ cup frozen raspberries
- ½ cup frozen blueberries
- ½ cup unsweetened almond milk
- ½ cup warm water
- 2 tablespoons almond butter
- 2 tablespoons pumpkin seeds
- 2 tablespoons broken pecans or walnuts

1. Place all ingredients in a blender. Blend until smooth. Add more liquid to adjust the thickness to your liking.

2. Serve immediately.

Makes 1 serving

Quick and Easy Breakfast Smoothie

INGREDIENTS
- 1 cup unsweetened plant-based milk
- 1 ripe banana, sliced
- ½ cup frozen raspberries
- ½ cup frozen blackberries
- 1 tablespoon coconut oil
- 1 teaspoon ground ginger
- ¼ cup pumpkin seeds

1. Place all ingredients in a blender. Blend until smooth. Add more liquid to adjust the thickness to your liking.

2. Serve immediately.

Makes 1 serving

Strawberry-Banana Protein Smoothie

INGREDIENTS
- 1 cup unsweetened almond milk
- 1 cup frozen strawberries
- 1 banana
- 1 scoop unsweetened plant-based protein powder
- 5 ice cubes
- ½ cup water (optional)

1. Place all ingredients in a blender. Blend until smooth. Add more liquid to adjust the thickness to your liking.

2. Serve immediately.

Makes 1 serving

Main Dishes

✓ Caramelized Cauliflower Steaks

INGREDIENTS
- 1 large head cauliflower, trimmed
- ½ cup extra-virgin olive oil
- Salt and freshly ground black pepper
- Lemon wedges

1. Preheat oven to 350 degrees. Use a sharp, heavy knife to cut cauliflower into 1-inch-thick steaks, starting at the center of cauliflower head and cutting through the stem end, from top to base. You should have four steak slices total. (Cook the extra pieces along with your steaks, as they are still great to eat.)

2. Lay the four steaks on a baking sheet, brush them with olive oil, and sprinkle with salt and pepper.

3. Heat the remainder of the oil in a large skillet over medium-high heat. Place as many of the steaks in the skillet as will comfortably fit. Fry for 2–3 minutes on each side or until golden brown and slightly softened; then return the steak to the baking sheet. Repeat until all the steaks are cooked.

4. Place the baking sheet in the oven and bake until the cauliflower steaks are tender, 10–15 minutes. Serve with lemon wedges, either hot or at room temperature.

Makes 4 servings

I like to whisk a little curry powder in the oil also. I serve these with a hearty green salad for a complete meal.

✓ Daniel Fast Marinara Sauce

INGREDIENTS
- 3 tablespoons olive oil
- 3 cups chopped yellow onion (about 3 medium)
- 3 teaspoons minced garlic (about 6 cloves)
- 2 teaspoons salt
- 2 teaspoons dried basil
- 1½ teaspoons dried oregano
- 1 teaspoon dried thyme
- 1 teaspoon freshly ground black pepper
- ½ teaspoon fennel seeds, crushed
- 2 tablespoons unsweetened balsamic vinegar
- 2 cups low-sodium vegetable broth
- 3 cans (28 ounces each) low-sodium crushed tomatoes

1. Heat oil in a large pot over medium heat. Add the onion and sauté for 4 minutes, stirring frequently. Gently stir in the minced garlic, salt, basil, oregano, thyme, black pepper, and fennel seeds; cook 1 minute, stirring constantly.

2. Add the vinegar and cook for 30 seconds; then add the vegetable broth and tomatoes. Bring to a simmer and cook uncovered over low heat for 55 minutes or until sauce thickens, stirring occasionally.

3. The sauce is now ready to use. To store in the freezer, cool the sauce and then ladle into plastic containers or zip-top plastic bags. Seal and freeze for up to four months. Consider freezing the sauce in one-cup measures, which would be two servings. That will allow you to use exactly as much as you want for future meals.

To boost the flavor of frozen sauce, add one-half teaspoon finely grated lemon rind or one teaspoon balsamic vinegar while reheating. Serve over whole wheat pasta, brown rice, slices of baked eggplant, or mixed with crumbled tofu and vegetables for a casserole.

Makes about 12 cups or 24 servings

Fajitas

INGREDIENTS
- 4 bell peppers, sliced
- 2 onions, sliced
- ½ pound mushrooms, sliced
- 2 serrano peppers, finely chopped
- 4 tablespoons olive oil, divided
- 2 teaspoons sugar-free seasoning salt
- ¼ teaspoon ground cumin
- Juice of 1 lime

Optional items to serve with filling:
- Whole wheat flour tortillas, warmed
- Diced tomatoes, pico de gallo, or salsa
- Freshly sliced avocado
- Cilantro
- Lime wedges
- Corn on the cob

1. In a small bowl, mix together the spices with the juice of 1 lime and 2 tablespoons of the olive oil; set aside.

2. Heat the remaining 2 tablespoons of olive oil in a large sauté pan over medium-high heat. Toss in the sliced bell peppers and onions; allow to cook until they begin to brown. Add the serrano peppers, sliced mushrooms, and the oil mixture and cook for 3–5 minutes.

3. Serve with warm tortillas and toppings of your choice.

Makes 4–6 servings

✓ Quinoa and Veggie Stir-Fry

INGREDIENTS
- 1 tablespoon olive oil
- ½ red bell pepper, chopped
- 2 cups packed baby spinach
- 1 cup cooked quinoa
- 2 cloves garlic, minced
- 1 teaspoon unsweetened soy sauce
- 1 teaspoon Asian chili-garlic paste

1. Heat oil in a skillet over medium-high heat. Stir-fry red pepper until just beginning to soften, about 5 minutes.

2. Stir in spinach, quinoa, garlic, soy sauce, and chili-garlic paste. Cook until heated through, about 3 minutes.

Makes 2 servings

Chinese Stir 'n Bake

INGREDIENTS
- 1 14-ounce package firm tofu, diced into bite-sized cubes
- 1 cup broccoli florets, stems removed
- 1 4-ounce package of sliced mushrooms, a variety of your choice
- ½ sweet onion, diced
- 1 cup Homemade Five-Spice Sauce (recipe follows)

1. Preheat oven to 400 degrees. While the oven is heating, prepare the tofu and the vegetables.

2. Place the tofu, broccoli, mushrooms, and onions in a large ovenproof baking dish. Drizzle with Homemade Five-Spice Sauce and then toss the vegetables to coat.

3. Cover the dish with foil and place in the preheated oven. Bake, covered, for 30–40 minutes.

Serve over whole grain noodles or brown rice.

Makes 4 servings

Homemade Five-Spice Sauce

INGREDIENTS
- 1 large sweet onion, finely chopped
- 2 tablespoons olive oil
- 6 cloves garlic, minced
- 2½ tablespoons gingerroot, minced
- 1½ cups vegetable broth
- 1 tablespoon unsweetened tomato paste
- ½ teaspoon freshly ground black pepper
- ¼ teaspoon red pepper flakes
- ¾ cup apple juice
- ¼ cup unsweetened soy sauce or tamari sauce
- 2 teaspoons Chinese five-spice powder

1. Heat the olive oil in a medium-sized saucepan over medium-high heat. Sauté the onion until it softens, about 4 minutes. Add the garlic and ginger and cook for another minute; then add the broth and continue cooking for another 5 minutes.

2. Spoon the onion-and-broth mixture into a blender. Cover and blend on low, increasing speed until mixture is smooth. You can also use an immersion blender right in the pot.

3. Return the mixture to the saucepan and add the remaining ingredients. Cook on low until it reduces slightly, about 10–15 minutes.

4. Store in a tightly sealed container in the refrigerator for up to 2 weeks.

Makes about 2½ cups

Fast and Easy Potato-Bean Casserole

INGREDIENTS
- 6 medium-sized new potatoes, cooked and cut into bite-sized pieces
- 1 tablespoon olive oil
- 1 clove garlic, minced
- 2 large yellow onions, chopped
- 1 tablespoon fresh oregano or 1 teaspoon dried oregano
- 1 can (15 ounces) diced tomatoes
- 1 can (15 ounces) chickpeas, drained and rinsed

- 1 can (15 ounces) white beans, drained and rinsed
- 10 Kalamata olives, cut in half lengthwise
- Salt and freshly ground black pepper to taste

1. Heat the oil in a large skillet over medium-high heat. Add the garlic, onion, and oregano. Reduce heat to medium and cook until the onion is soft and translucent, about 10 minutes.

2. Stir in the tomatoes, chickpeas, and white beans. Simmer until the liquid starts to evaporate and thicken, about 5 minutes. Add the potatoes and olives; cover and cook for about 10 more minutes, stirring occasionally.

3. Season with salt and pepper before serving.

Makes 6 servings

Sweet Potato Curry

INGREDIENTS
- 1 pound sweet potatoes (about 3 medium), peeled, cooked, and diced into bite-sized pieces
- 1 tablespoon olive oil
- 2 large onions, chopped
- 2 tablespoons grated fresh gingerroot
- 1 tablespoon ground cumin
- 2 teaspoons curry powder
- 1 can (15 ounces) diced tomatoes
- 2 cans (15 ounces each) chickpeas, drained and rinsed
- Juice of 1 lemon

1. Heat the oil in a large skillet over medium-high heat. Add the onions, ginger, cumin, and curry powder; reduce heat to medium and stir the ingredients to blend the spices with the onions. Continue to cook until the onion is soft and translucent, about 10 minutes.

2. Add the tomatoes and chickpeas and stir to blend well. Reduce heat to low; cover and simmer for 5–7 minutes.

3. Add the diced sweet potatoes and gently stir to combine all the ingredients. Add the lemon juice just before serving.

Makes 4 servings

Pasta with Tomatoes, Olives, and Capers

INGREDIENTS
- 4 cups hot cooked whole-grain penne pasta
- 4 cups halved cherry tomatoes (about 2 pints)
- ⅓ cup thinly sliced fresh basil
- ¼ cup chopped pitted Kalamata olives
- 2 tablespoons capers
- 2 tablespoons extra-virgin olive oil
- ¾ teaspoon salt
- ½ teaspoon crushed red pepper
- ½ teaspoon freshly ground black pepper
- 2 cloves garlic, minced

1. Slice tomatoes and basil.

2. Prepare pasta according to package directions. Drain.

3. Mix all the ingredients together and serve. How easy is that!

Makes 4 servings

Tofu Stir-Fry with Cashews and Baby Bok Choy

You can serve this tofu stir-fry over rice, quinoa, whole-grain noodles, or even over a bed of spinach greens.

INGREDIENTS
- 2 tablespoons unsweetened soy sauce, divided
- 1 tablespoon rice wine vinegar
- 1 tablespoon cornstarch
- 1 14-ounce block extra-firm tofu, pressed and cut into bite-sized cubes or strips
- 2 tablespoons toasted sesame oil
- 2 tablespoons olive oil
- ½ of a large sweet onion, chopped
- 4 cloves garlic, minced
- 2-inch piece gingerroot, minced
- 1 teaspoon apple juice
- 6 bunches baby bok choy, chopped into bite-sized pieces

- ½ cup roasted, unsalted cashews, coarsely chopped
- 1 bunch green onions, chopped

1. Whisk together 1 tablespoon of soy sauce, vinegar, and cornstarch in a large bowl. Add the tofu pieces and gently toss to coat.

2. Heat the sesame oil in a large skillet or wok over medium high. Add the tofu and all of the sauce to the pan. Cook, stirring frequently, until the liquid almost completely evaporates and the tofu begins to brown, about 10 minutes. Transfer back to the bowl and set aside.

3. Using the same pan, heat the olive oil over medium-high heat. Add the onion and garlic and cook until the onion softens.

4. Add the gingerroot, the other tablespoon of soy sauce, the apple juice, and the baby bok choy, stir-frying until the green part of the bok choy begins to soften and turns bright green.

5. Return the tofu to the pan and gently stir until all the ingredients are heated.

6. Transfer to a warmed serving bowl and sprinkle with cashews and green onions. Serve hot.

Makes 4 servings

Savory Stir-Fry Tofu

INGREDIENTS

For the stir-fry:
- 1 14-ounce package firm or extra firm tofu, well-drained and cut into bite-sized cubes
- 2 cups roughly chopped green beans
- 1 carrot, diced
- 1 red bell pepper, diced
- 2 tablespoons sesame oil

For the sauce:
- ¼ cup unsweetened soy sauce or tamari sauce
- 1 tablespoon grated fresh gingerroot

- 2 tablespoons apple juice
- 1 tablespoon cornstarch

1. Preheat oven to 400 degrees.

2. Arrange the cubed tofu on a baking sheet lightly coated with cooking spray or lined with parchment paper. Bake for 15 minutes. Flip the cubes and return to the oven for 15–20 more minutes to dry out the tofu and help give it a meat-like texture. You can adjust this baking time to give the tofu the texture and dryness you prefer.

3. When the tofu has browned, remove from the oven. Allow to cool and continue drying while you prepare the remainder of your ingredients.

4. In a small mixing bowl, whisk together all of the sauce ingredients and set aside.

5. Add the sesame oil to a large skillet, coating the bottom of the pan and heating over medium-high heat. Add the beans, carrots, and bell pepper and toss to coat. Cook for 5–7 minutes, stirring often.

6. Add the sauce and stir until it begins to bubble and slightly thicken; add the tofu and gently stir to coat.

7. Cook the mixture for 3–5 minutes, stirring frequently. When the vegetables are cooked to your liking, remove from heat.

8. Serve alone or over brown rice for a more filling meal.

Makes 2–3 servings

Designer Meal in a Bowl

Use your imagination. Let your bowl be like a blank canvas, with you as the designer. Consider what you like and what you have available; then create your uniquely designed meal in a bowl.

INGREDIENTS
- 2 cups brown rice, cooked
- 1 can (15 ounces) black beans, drained and rinsed
- 1 can (15 ounces) diced tomatoes
- 2 tablespoons unsweetened soy sauce

- 1 teaspoon apple cider vinegar
- 1 teaspoon chili powder
- 1 avocado, diced
- Seasonings and toppings to taste (see following)

1. Prepare brown rice using your preferred method (stove top or rice cooker).

2. In a medium saucepan over medium heat, stir together the beans, tomatoes, soy sauce, chili powder, and any other spices and seasonings you choose. Heat for about 15 minutes, or until it's hot and the liquid has slightly reduced. Remove from heat and gently stir in the apple cider vinegar.

3. While the beans and tomatoes are heating, spoon 1 cup of the hot, cooked brown rice into each of two individual serving bowls. Spoon the hot bean-tomato mixture over the rice, and then top with the diced avocado. Serve immediately.

Makes 2 servings

To vary your designer meal in a bowl, use any of the following for a base (or come up with your own idea):
- brown rice
- whole-grain couscous
- quinoa
- whole-grain pasta

Be creative with your hot mixture concoction, depending on what ingredients you have on hand, for instance:
- fresh or frozen corn or peas
- green or red bell peppers
- chickpeas, kidney beans, or white beans
- greens, including kale or spinach
- onions, diced or sliced
- tofu diced into cubes

Then add your final topping for a special kick of flavor and color:
- chopped green onion
- jalapeño slices
- Kalamata olives

- sunflower seeds
- toasted nuts

You can also get creative with the sauce for your designer bowl. The basic recipe uses the juice from the tomatoes and the soy sauce to create a sauce, but be creative and come up with your own ideas. For example, skip the soy sauce and add cumin instead. Toss in corn with the black beans and go a little more Latin.

Letting other family members join you in the creative process can be fun and may also encourage them to eat new and different foods.

Easy Red Beans and Rice

INGREDIENTS
- 1 medium onion, chopped
- ½ green pepper, chopped
- 2 ribs celery, chopped
- 3 cloves garlic, minced
- 2 tablespoons water
- 3 cans (15 ounces each) red beans, drained and rinsed
- 1 can (15 ounces) roasted tomatoes
- 1 teaspoon dried thyme
- 1 teaspoon dried oregano
- 1 teaspoon smoked paprika
- 1 teaspoon salt (optional or to taste)
- ½ teaspoon freshly ground black pepper
- ¼ to 1 teaspoon cayenne pepper (to taste)
- 2 teaspoons hot sauce, plus more to serve
- 2 cups cooked brown rice

1. Heat a large, nonstick pot over medium-high heat. Add the water and the onions, green pepper, celery, and garlic to the pot. Cook until softened, stirring occasionally, 6–10 minutes.

2. When the vegetables are softened, stir in the beans, tomatoes, thyme, oregano, and paprika. Cover tightly and then reduce heat to very low. Cook for about 30 minutes, stirring every 5–10 minutes. Add water as needed to keep beans moist but not soupy.

3. Just before serving, sprinkle with salt, black pepper, cayenne pepper, and hot sauce to your desired taste. (Remember, add just a little at a time as you can always add more but you can't take it away.)

4. To serve family style, place the hot brown rice in a large serving bowl and then pour the hot bean and tomato mixture over the top. You can also portion brown rice into individual serving bowls and top with the bean and tomato mixture. Serve with hot sauce for those who might want more spice.

Red Beans and Rice

INGREDIENTS
- 1 tablespoon olive oil
- 2 large cloves garlic, minced
- 1 large red onion, chopped
- 1 stalk celery, chopped
- 1 green bell pepper, chopped
- 2 cans (15 ounces each) red kidney beans, undrained
- 1 teaspoon onion powder
- 1 teaspoon salt
- ¼ teaspoon ground black pepper
- 1 tablespoon hot sauce
- 2½ cups vegetable broth
- 2 cups cooked brown rice
- 1 tablespoon minced fresh cilantro leaves

1. Heat the olive oil over medium-high heat in a large saucepan. Sauté the garlic, onion, celery, and bell pepper until tender. Stir in the kidney beans, onion powder, salt, pepper, and hot sauce; reduce heat to low and let mixture simmer slowly.

2. Add the vegetable broth and bring to a boil. Stir in the cooked brown rice; remove from heat and let stand for 5 minutes.

3. Serve garnished with cilantro.

Makes 6 servings

Bean and Garden Burgers

Because of the Daniel Fast restrictions, bean burgers cannot be eaten with traditional buns. Try them on their own, topped with sautéed vegetables, or with chapatis (see recipe on page 202).

Black Bean and Quinoa Veggie Burgers

INGREDIENTS
- 3 cups water, divided
- ½ cup quinoa
- 1 small yellow onion, finely chopped
- 6 oil-packed sun-dried tomatoes, drained and finely chopped (reserve the oil)
- 1½ cups well-cooked black beans, or one can (14 ounces) black beans, drained, divided
- 2 cloves garlic, minced
- 2 teaspoons unsweetened steak seasoning
- Salt to taste

1. Combine 1½ cups salted water and the quinoa in a small saucepan. Bring to a boil, cover, and reduce heat to medium-low. Simmer for about 20 minutes or until all the liquid is absorbed.

2. While the quinoa cooks, place the chopped onion and sun-dried tomatoes in a medium nonstick skillet. Cook over medium heat 3–4 minutes or until the onion is softened and translucent. If necessary, add a bit more of the reserved oil to make sure the onion doesn't stick.

3. Add ¾ cup black beans to the skillet along with the garlic, steak seasoning, and 1½ cups water; simmer 9–11 minutes or until most of liquid is absorbed.

4. Place the bean-onion mixture into a food processor along with ¾ cup cooked quinoa. Process the mixture until smooth but not pureed.

5. Transfer the bean-quinoa mixture to a medium bowl and stir in the remaining quinoa and the remaining ¾ cup black beans. Season with salt and pepper and allow the mixture to cool.

6. Preheat the oven to 350 degrees. Coat a baking sheet with olive oil or cooking spray. Separate the mixture into 8 equal portions (about ½ cup each) and then shape the portions into patties. Place each patty onto the prepared baking sheet.

7. Bake 20 minutes, or until the patties are brown and crisp on top. Carefully turn the patties with a spatula and bake 10 minutes more or until both sides are crisp and brown.

8. Serve with side dishes and a salad for a complete and nutritious meal.

Makes 8 servings

Quick and Easy Bean Burgers

INGREDIENTS
- 2 cups well-cooked beans (black, red, or white) or one 14-ounce can of beans, drained (reserve some liquid)
- 1 medium yellow onion, quartered
- ½ cup rolled oats
- ½ cup cooked brown rice
- 1 tablespoon chili powder
- Salt and freshly ground pepper
- Olive oil, as needed

1. Place the beans, onion, rolled oats, rice, chili powder, salt, and pepper in a food processor.

2. Pulse the ingredients to combine, making sure they remain chunky and not pureed. Add a little water or reserved bean liquid if necessary.

3. Separate the mixture into equal amounts; with wet hands shape the mixture into patties.

4. Coat a nonstick skillet with olive oil; heat over medium and add the burgers. Cook until nicely browned on one side (about 5 minutes) and then carefully turn to brown the other side (about 5 more minutes). Cook until patties are well-heated and firm.

5. Serve with side dishes and a salad for a complete and nutritious meal.

Makes 4–6 servings

✓ Spicy Vegetable Burgers

INGREDIENTS

- 2 pounds fresh kale, collards, spinach, or mustard greens, washed and roughly chopped
- 2 cups well-cooked or canned beans, well drained
- 4–5 tablespoons extra-virgin olive oil, divided
- 1 medium sweet potato or yam, peeled and grated (about 1 cup)
- Salt and pepper
- ½ cup crushed whole wheat matzo crackers
- ½ teaspoon ground cinnamon
- ¼ teaspoon ground nutmeg

1. Heat the olive oil over medium heat in a large sauté pan. Add the greens and cover the pan; cook for about 5 minutes or until completely wilted.

2. Place the beans in a large bowl and mash with a fork. Add the greens and mix thoroughly.

3. Heat 2 tablespoons of the olive oil in a large skillet over medium heat. Add the sweet potato and season with salt and pepper. Cook the potato, stirring frequently, until it begins to soften, about 5 minutes. Add the crushed matzo, cinnamon, and nutmeg; stir and cook for another minute.

4. Combine the bean mixture with the sweet potato mixture. If the mixture is too wet, add a little more crushed matzo cracker. Adjust seasoning to taste. Divide the mixture into 4–6 equal portions and form into patties.

5. Heat 2 tablespoons of olive oil in the skillet over medium heat. When the oil is heated, carefully add the patties to the pan, cooking until browned on one side (about 5 minutes). Carefully turn the patties and cook the other side until browned and firm.

6. Serve with side dishes and a salad for a nutritious meal.

Makes 4–6 servings

Sweet Vegan Burgers

INGREDIENTS
- 1 can (15 ounces) chickpeas, drained and rinsed
- 1 can (15 ounces) whole kernel sweet corn, drained
- ½ cup coarsely chopped cilantro
- ½ teaspoon paprika
- ½ teaspoon ground coriander
- ½ teaspoon ground cumin
- Zest of 1 lemon
- 3 heaped tablespoons whole wheat flour, plus extra for dusting
- Sea salt
- Grape seed oil (grape seed oil works well with high heat)

1. Place the chickpeas, corn, cilantro, paprika, coriander, cumin, and lemon zest in a food processor. Pulse until smooth but still slightly chunky.

2. On a flour-dusted surface, divide the mixture and shape into four patties, similar to the size of a typical meat patty. Set on a tray and place in the refrigerator for about 30 minutes so the patties will be firm.

3. Heat a little grape seed oil in a large frying pan over medium heat. Add the patties and cook for a total of 10–12 minutes, or until golden and cooked through, turning halfway through cooking time. Serve hot.

Makes 4 servings

Soups and Stews

✓ Basic Vegetable Soup

INGREDIENTS
- 2 tablespoons olive oil
- 2 medium yellow onions, chopped
- 2 stalks celery, chopped
- 2 teaspoons Italian herbs
- Kosher salt and freshly ground black pepper to taste
- 3 cans (15 ounces each) vegetable broth
- 1 large can (28 ounces) diced tomatoes, including juice
- 1 tablespoon unsweetened tomato paste
- 3 cups water
- 8 cups fresh or frozen mixed vegetables, such as carrots, corn, green beans, peas, potatoes, and squash (You can also include canned beans such as kidney, pinto, or black beans.)

1. Heat the oil in a large soup pot over medium heat. Add the onions, celery, and Italian herbs. Cook, stirring frequently, until the onions are translucent, 5–8 minutes.

2. Add the broth, tomatoes and their juice, tomato paste, and 3 cups water to the pot and bring to a boil. Reduce the heat to a simmer and cook uncovered for 20 minutes.

3. Next add the vegetables to the pot and return to a simmer; cook uncovered until the vegetables are tender, 20–25 minutes.

4. Season with salt and pepper to taste and serve.

Makes 8 servings

Moroccan Stew

INGREDIENTS
- 2 teaspoons olive oil
- 2 medium onions, chopped
- ½ cup unsweetened peanut butter
- 3 sweet potatoes, peeled and cubed into bite-sized pieces
- 1 teaspoon ground cumin
- ¼ teaspoon cinnamon
- ¼ teaspoon curry powder
- ½ teaspoon freshly ground black pepper
- ¼ teaspoon kosher salt
- 2 cans (15 ounces each) chickpeas, drained and rinsed
- 4 cups vegetable broth
- 1 can (28 ounces) diced tomatoes, including juice
- 1 bunch fresh kale, chopped
- Italian parsley sprigs for garnish

1. Heat the oil in a large soup pot over medium-high heat. Add the onion and sauté until lightly browned, 7 minutes.

2. Add the peanut butter, sweet potato, cumin, cinnamon, curry powder, black pepper, salt, chickpeas, vegetable broth, tomatoes with their juice, and chopped kale. Bring to a boil; reduce heat and simmer, uncovered, 30 minutes or until sweet potato is tender.

3. Serve and garnish with parsley, if desired.

Makes 8 servings

Greek Lentil Soup

INGREDIENTS
- 1 cup brown lentils, rinsed
- ¼ cup olive oil
- 1 tablespoon minced garlic
- 1 medium yellow onion, minced
- 1 large carrot, peeled and chopped
- 2 stalks celery, chopped into small dice
- 1 quart water
- 1 teaspoon Italian herbs
- 1 tablespoon unsweetened tomato paste
- Kosher salt and freshly ground black pepper to taste
- Olive oil for serving, if desired

1. Place the lentils in a large saucepan; add enough water to cover by 1 inch. Bring the water to a boil and cook until the lentils begin to soften, about 10 minutes; drain.

2. While the lentils are cooking, heat the olive oil in a saucepan over medium heat. Add the garlic, onion, carrot, and celery; cook and stir until the onion has softened and turned translucent, 5–6 minutes.

3. Add the lentils to the onion mixture in a saucepan along with 1 quart water and Italian herbs; bring to a boil, then reduce the heat to medium-low. Cover and simmer for 10 minutes.

4. Stir in the tomato paste and season with salt and pepper. Cover and simmer, stirring occasionally, until the lentils are completely soft, 30–40 minutes. Add additional water if the soup becomes too thick.

5. To serve, drizzle each portion with 1 teaspoon olive oil.

Makes 4 servings

Northern Africa Spicy Soup

INGREDIENTS
- 1 tablespoon olive oil
- 3 medium carrots, peeled and finely chopped
- 2 stalks celery, finely diced
- 1 large yellow onion, finely chopped
- 2 cloves garlic, minced
- 1 teaspoon ground cumin
- 1 teaspoon ground ginger
- 1 teaspoon coriander
- ½ teaspoon ground turmeric
- ¼ teaspoon ground cinnamon
- 1 teaspoon kosher salt
- One can (28 ounces) diced tomatoes, with juice
- Two cans (15 ounces each) chickpeas, drained and rinsed
- 1 cup dried brown lentils
- ½ cup whole grain orzo pasta
- 4 cups vegetable broth
- Juice of ½ lemon
- ¼ cup finely chopped cilantro leaves

1. Heat the olive oil in a large pot over medium heat. Add the carrots, celery, and onion and cook, stirring occasionally, until soft, 10–12 minutes. Gently stir in the garlic, cumin, ginger, coriander, turmeric, cinnamon, and salt; cook, stirring often, for 1½–2 minutes.

2. Add the diced tomatoes and continue to cook, stirring up any browned bits from the bottom of the pot, until the mixture begins to thicken, 5–7 minutes.

3. Stir in the chickpeas, lentils, and orzo along with the vegetable broth. Bring to a simmer over high heat and then reduce the heat to medium-low and cook until the lentils are tender, 15–20 minutes.

4. Just before serving the hot soup, stir in the lemon juice and most of the cilantro. Sprinkle with the remaining cilantro for garnish.

Makes 4 servings

Susan's Vegetarian Chili

This recipe was published in *The Daniel Fast: Feed Your Soul, Strengthen Your Spirit, and Renew Your Body,* and since then I have received countless messages about how much people like it because of its ease, low cost, and rich flavor and textures. It's also an easy recipe to modify to your own liking or based on what you have in your pantry.

INGREDIENTS
- 2 medium green peppers, chopped
- 1 medium yellow onion, chopped
- 1 zucchini, sliced
- 1 yellow squash, sliced
- 2 tablespoons olive oil
- 2 tablespoons chili powder
- ¾ teaspoon salt
- ¼ teaspoon ground red pepper
- 2 cups corn kernels, fresh or frozen
- 2 cans (15 ounces each) tomatoes, including juice
- 2 cans (15 ounces each) pinto beans, including liquid
- 2 cans (15 ounces each) black beans, including liquid
- 1 can (4 ounces) mild green chilies
- 1 can (4 ounces) unsweetened tomato paste

1. Chop the peppers and onions and sauté in oil. Add the sliced squashes, chili powder, salt, ground red pepper, and corn.

2. When all the vegetables are softened but still firm, add the tomatoes, all the beans, the green chilies, and the tomato paste; stir until just blended.

3. Bring to a boil and then reduce the heat. Let simmer for 20 minutes, stirring occasionally to prevent sticking.

4. Serve. (This recipe also freezes well.)

Makes 6 generous servings

Slow Cooker Vegetable Lentil Soup

INGREDIENTS
- 2 cups brown lentils, rinsed
- 1 can (15 ounces) diced tomatoes, including juice
- 3 carrots, cut into ¼-inch rounds

- 3 stalks celery, cut into ¼-inch pieces
- 1 medium yellow onion, finely chopped
- 2 cloves garlic, minced
- ½ teaspoon Italian herbs
- 5 cups vegetable broth
- 2 cups water
- Kosher salt and freshly ground black pepper to taste
- ¼ cup chopped fresh Italian parsley

1. Place the lentils, tomatoes, carrots, celery, onion, garlic, Italian herbs, broth, and 2 cups of water in the slow cooker. Cover and cook on low until lentils and vegetables are tender, about 6 hours.

2. Transfer 2 cups of the soup to a blender. Let cool for 5 minutes and then puree the mixture; return pureed soup to the slow cooker.

3. Season the soup with salt and pepper; garnish with parsley and serve.

Makes 4 servings

Vegetable Rice Stew

INGREDIENTS
- 1 medium yellow onion, coarsely chopped
- 3 carrots, cut into ¼-inch rounds
- 3 yellow potatoes, diced into bite-sized pieces
- 1 parsnip, diced into bite-sized pieces
- 1 turnip, diced into bite-sized pieces
- 1 teaspoon ground black pepper
- 1 teaspoon ground cumin
- 1 teaspoon kosher salt
- 2½ cups water
- ½ cup cooked brown rice or barley
- ¼ cup chopped Italian parsley, for garnish

1. In a large pot over medium-high heat, combine onion, carrots, potatoes, parsnip, turnip, pepper, cumin, salt, and water. Boil until vegetables are tender, about 30 minutes, adding more water if necessary.

2. Just before serving, stir in the cooked brown rice or barley; garnish with parsley and serve.

Makes 4 servings

Side Dishes

Fast, Easy, and Tasty Black Beans

INGREDIENTS
- 1 can (15 ounces) black beans, undrained
- 1 small onion, chopped
- 1 clove garlic, minced
- ½ teaspoon cumin
- Salt to taste
- 1 tablespoon chopped fresh cilantro

1. In a medium saucepan over medium heat, combine beans, onion, garlic, cumin, and salt. Bring to a boil; reduce heat to medium-low and continue to simmer for 4–5 more minutes.

2. Adjust seasoning and then garnish with cilantro. Serve.

Makes 4 servings

✓ Cauliflower "Rice"

INGREDIENTS
- 1 head cauliflower, cut into florets
- 2 tablespoons water
- 1 fresh lime, zest and juice
- ½ cup chopped cilantro
- 1 tablespoon olive oil

1. Place the cauliflower in a food processor and pulse until it looks similar to rice. (You can also use a food grater for this step.)

2. Place the cauliflower in a saucepan, add the water, and heat over medium heat until the cauliflower is tender, 5–7 minutes.

3. Meanwhile, zest the lime into a small bowl and then squeeze the juice from the lime into the same bowl. Stir in the cilantro and olive oil and blend.

4. When the cauliflower is tender, pour the lime and cilantro mixture into the pan and gently stir to blend.

5. Serve hot as a side dish.

Makes 4 servings

Cinnamon-Roasted Butternut Squash

INGREDIENTS
- 1 large butternut squash, peeled, seeded, and cut into bite-sized cubes
- 2 tablespoons olive oil
- ½ teaspoon ground cinnamon
- 1 teaspoon kosher salt
- Dash of cayenne (optional)

1. Preheat oven to 425 degrees. Line two large baking sheets with aluminum foil.

2. Place the squash cubes in a large bowl and set aside.

3. Using a small bowl, whisk together the olive oil, cinnamon, salt, and cayenne pepper until well blended. Drizzle the oil mixture over the squash cubes and toss until the cubes are all coated.

4. Arrange the squash cubes on the prepared baking pans; place in the oven and roast for a total of 40–45 minutes. Halfway through the cooking time, rotate the pans to promote even cooking. Continue to roast until the cubes are browned and the centers are softened.

5. Serve as a side dish on its own or along with brown rice or quinoa and other roasted vegetables.

Makes 4 servings

Super-Easy Homemade Applesauce

INGREDIENTS
- 3 pounds Granny Smith apples, peeled and cut into large chunks (or use the apple variety of your choice)
- ½ cup apple juice
- 1 tablespoon fresh lemon juice
- 1 large cinnamon stick or ½ teaspoon ground cinnamon (or to taste)
- ¼ teaspoon ground nutmeg

1. In a large pot over medium heat, combine the apples, apple juice, lemon juice, and cinnamon. Cover and simmer until the apples become tender but not mushy, 20–25 minutes.

2. Remove the cinnamon stick if you used one. Then use an immersion blender right in the pot to pulse the apples to applesauce consistency. You can also transfer the apples and the juice to a food processor and pulse the contents into a smooth consistency.

3. Add the nutmeg and serve warm, or store in the fridge to serve cold later. Freezes well.

Makes 6 servings

✓ Quick 'n Easy Quinoa Side Dish

INGREDIENTS
- 1 tablespoon olive oil
- 1 cup uncooked quinoa
- 2 cups low-sodium vegetable broth
- 2 teaspoons minced garlic
- 2 tablespoons chopped fresh parsley
- ½ tablespoon chopped fresh thyme
- ¼ teaspoon salt
- 1 small onion, finely chopped
- Juice of 1 lemon, to personal taste

1. Heat the olive oil in a saucepan over medium heat. Add the quinoa and toast, stirring occasionally, until lightly browned, about 5 minutes.

2. Stir in the broth and bring to a boil. Reduce to a simmer, cover, and cook until the quinoa is tender, about 15 minutes.

3. Meanwhile, combine the garlic, parsley, thyme, salt, and onion in a bowl. When the quinoa is ready, add it to the bowl and gently stir to combine. Sprinkle with lemon juice to taste.

Makes 4 servings

Quinoa with Toasted Nuts

INGREDIENTS
- 1 cup uncooked quinoa, rinsed and drained
- 3 teaspoons olive oil, divided
- 2 tablespoons finely chopped shallots
- 1 tablespoon minced garlic
- 1¼ cups low-sodium vegetable broth
- ¼ teaspoon kosher salt
- ¼ cup pine nuts
- ¼ cup chopped fresh Italian parsley
- 2 tablespoons chopped fresh chives
- ¼ teaspoon freshly ground black pepper

1. Heat a large saucepan over medium-high heat. Add 2 teaspoons of the olive oil to the pan and swirl to coat. Add the shallots and sauté until tender, about 1 minute. Add the minced garlic and cook 1 minute, stirring constantly.

2. Next, add the quinoa to the pot and cook 2 minutes, stirring frequently. Stir in the vegetable stock and kosher salt and bring to a boil. Cover and reduce heat; simmer until liquid is absorbed and quinoa is tender, 12–13 minutes.

3. While quinoa cooks, heat a large nonstick skillet over medium heat. Add the pine nuts to the pan and cook, stirring frequently, until they are lightly browned, about 3 minutes.

4. Combine the quinoa mixture with the roasted pine nuts. Sprinkle with the remaining olive oil, parsley, chives, and pepper.

Makes 4 servings

✓ Spaghetti Squash

INGREDIENTS
- 1 spaghetti squash
- 2 tablespoons olive oil
- 1 teaspoon dried oregano
- 1 teaspoon kosher salt

1. Preheat oven to 375 degrees.

2. Place the whole spaghetti squash in a baking dish. Bake for 45–60 minutes or until a sharp knife can easily pierce the squash.

3. Remove the squash from the oven. Using a sharp knife, cut the squash in half length-wise. Scoop out and discard the seeds and the surrounding stringy fibers.

4. Allow the squash to cool for a few minutes. Then, using a dinner fork, "comb" the flesh of the squash so that it separates into spaghetti-like strings. Discard the outer shell.

5. Heat the oil in a large skillet. Add the spaghetti squash, oregano, and salt. Toss until all ingredients are mixed; serve.

Makes 4 servings

✓ Easy Roasted Vegetables

Here is an easy way to roast vegetables for a side dish, to use in recipes, or to eat as a snack. While the vegetables take a while to roast, they are quick and simple to prepare.

INGREDIENTS
- Canola or olive oil
- Assorted vegetables, such as yams or sweet potatoes, carrots, turnips, beets, cauliflower, onions, potatoes, or squash
- Seasonings, such as rosemary, basil, parsley, marjoram, salt, and pepper
- Broth, apple juice, or Italian dressing (to taste)

1. Preheat oven to 400 degrees. Line a jellyroll pan with foil, and coat the foil with canola or olive oil cooking spray. Cut your vegetables into small chunks.

2. Add vegetables in a single layer to the foil-lined pan. Either spray the top with cooking spray or drizzle with a bit of canola or olive oil (no more than a teaspoon of oil for every cup of vegetables). If you use oil, toss the veggies in the pan to coat.

3. Sprinkle on any desired seasonings, such as rosemary, basil, parsley, marjoram, salt, and pepper. Coat the tops of your veggies again with canola or olive oil cooking spray, if desired, especially if you didn't drizzle with oil in step 2.

4. Bake until veggies are lightly browned and tender. If your vegetables look like they are starting to dry out during the roasting period, drizzle some broth, apple juice, or low-fat Italian dressing or vinaigrette over the top. Different vegetables require different cooking times. Check your roasted vegetables after 25–30 minutes, turn them over with a spatula, and then cook until they're tender and nicely browned around some of the edges (about 25–30 minutes more).

A serving is ½ cup roasted vegetables.

Sweet Potato Fries

INGREDIENTS
- 4 medium sweet potatoes, unpeeled
- 4 tablespoons olive oil
- 2 teaspoons ground coriander
- 1 teaspoon kosher salt

1. Preheat the oven to 400 degrees.

2. Cut each sweet potato lengthwise into 8 wedges.

3. Place the sweet potato wedges in a large bowl. Drizzle the olive oil over the potatoes and then sprinkle with the coriander. Using your hands, toss the wedges until they are well coated.

4. Line a baking sheet with parchment paper. Arrange the sweet potato wedges so they are flat on the pan and are not touching each other. Roast for about 25 minutes or until tender.

5. Remove from the oven and sprinkle with the kosher salt.

Makes 4 servings

✓ Easy Quinoa Side Dish

INGREDIENTS
- 3 cups quinoa, rinsed and thoroughly drained
- 3 cloves garlic, minced
- ½ of a yellow onion, chopped
- 2–3 tablespoons olive oil
- 5 cups vegetable stock
- Salt and pepper

1. Heat a large saucepan over medium-high heat. Add the quinoa and toast it, stirring frequently until the quinoa makes popping sounds, 5–7 minutes. Transfer the quinoa to a bowl and set aside.

2. Using the same pan, heat the oil over medium-high heat. Sauté the garlic and onion until softened, 3–5 minutes. Add the quinoa to the mixture and stir until combined.

3. Add the vegetable stock. Bring to a boil, then reduce to low; cover and simmer for 13–15 minutes or until you see the little circles separating from the grains. Salt and pepper to taste.

4. Serve hot. Refrigerate or freeze the leftovers.

Makes 12 servings

Rice and Whole Grains

Brown Rice

If you are not accustomed to cooking brown rice, know that it does not cook the same way as the white variety (where the bran and the germ parts of the grain have been removed). Generally, brown rice takes longer to cook and also uses more water. I cook my rice using an inexpensive rice cooker I purchased about 10 years ago for $15. This little workhorse cooks the rice to perfection in about 45 minutes.

INGREDIENTS
- 1 cup brown rice, rinsed
- 2½ cups water
- ½ teaspoon salt

1. Place the rice, water, and salt in a large saucepan with a tightly fitting lid. Bring the rice to a boil and then cover the pan and reduce the heat; simmer for 40–50 minutes.

2. When the rice is done, keep covered and let it rest for 5 minutes.

3. Serve or use in a recipe calling for cooked rice.

Makes 3 cups rice

Freezing Cooked Rice

To save time, cook a large batch of brown rice and freeze the extra. (This method also works for other grains, including barley, bulgur wheat, farro, millet, and quinoa.)

1. Cook the brown rice in your rice cooker or follow the instructions above to cook on the stove top.

2. Prepare large baking pans by running them under water and then shaking off the excess water. Don't dry the pan. This step keeps the cooked rice from sticking to the pan.

3. Spread the cooked rice on the pans in a single layer (as well as you can) and allow to cool for about 10 minutes.

4. Scoop the cooled rice into plastic freezer bags that you've dated and labeled Cooked Brown Rice. To portion the rice in the bags, use a 1-cup measuring cup rinsed in cold water. Scoop the rice into the cup and transfer to the plastic freezer bags.

5. Seal the bags and lay them flat in your freezer. Keeps for several weeks.

6. To use the rice, place the frozen rice in a microwave-safe bowl; cover and heat for 1 minute on high power. Now it's ready to eat or use in a recipe calling for cooked rice.

Barley

Barley is a nutritious and hearty whole grain that is inexpensive and easy to prepare.

INGREDIENTS
- 1 cup barley
- 2½ cups water or broth

1. Place the water and the barley in a large pot with a tightly fitting cover; bring to a boil, then reduce heat to a simmer. Cover and cook until tender and most of the liquid has been absorbed, 40–50 minutes.

2. Let stand 5 minutes and then serve or add to other recipes.

Makes 3–3½ cups

Bulgur Wheat

Bulgur is wheat that's been parboiled, dried, and cracked into bits. It cooks fast and has a pleasant flavor. You can use it to increase the protein value of salads, soups, casseroles, and smoothies. Bulgur wheat is available in most supermarkets, or you can find it at your local health food store.

INGREDIENTS
- 1½ cups medium-grain bulgur wheat
- 3 cups water

1. Combine the bulgur and the water in a medium saucepan with a tightly fitting lid. Bring to a boil, cover, reduce heat, and simmer for 10–12 minutes or until the bulgur wheat is tender.

2. Drain any excess liquid and then use in a recipe of your choice, sprinkle over salads, or add to soup.

Makes 5 cups

Quinoa

Quinoa has stormed onto the health scene over the last several years, and for good reason. The whole grain has all the amino acids to make it a complete protein, plus it's easy to cook and very nutritious.

INGREDIENTS
- 1 cup uncooked quinoa
- 3 cups water or broth

1. Bring the quinoa and water or broth to a boil in a medium saucepan. Reduce heat to low, cover, and simmer until tender and most of the liquid has been absorbed, 15–20 minutes.

2. Fluff with a fork and serve or use as an ingredient in a recipe.

Makes 3 cups

Farro

Farro is a spelt wheat grain with ancient roots in Italy. The grain has a nutty flavor and can be eaten plain, but it is most often used in grain salads or added to soups.

INGREDIENTS
- 1 cup farro
- 3 cups water or stock

Here are two ways to cook farro:

Traditional
1. Rinse and drain the farro before placing it in a pot with a tight-fitting lid. Add enough water or stock to cover and bring to a boil over medium-high heat. Reduce heat to medium-low and simmer 30 minutes; drain off any excess water.

2. Serve or use in a recipe.

For quick-cooking farro
1. Cover the farro with water and soak in the refrigerator overnight; drain. Place in a pot and add water or stock to cover. Then bring to a boil; reduce heat to medium-low and simmer 10 minutes. Drain off any excess water.

2. Serve or use in a recipe.

Makes 4 servings (about 2 cups)

Salads

✓ Asian-Style Coleslaw Salad

INGREDIENTS
- 3 cups chopped coleslaw cabbage (available in the produce section)
- 1 bunch radishes, julienned
- ⅓ cup chopped green onions
- ⅓ cup chopped fresh cilantro
- 3 tablespoons unsweetened soy sauce
- 1 tablespoon apple cider vinegar
- 1 tablespoon olive oil
- 2 teaspoons grated fresh gingerroot
- 1 teaspoon fresh lime juice
- Dash of red pepper
- Toasted sesame seeds for garnish

1. In a large bowl, toss together the coleslaw, radishes, green onions, and cilantro; set aside.

2. In a small bowl, whisk together the soy sauce, vinegar, oil, ginger, lime juice, and red pepper.

3. Pour the dressing over the coleslaw mixture and combine until evenly coated.

4. Garnish with the toasted sesame seeds and serve.

Makes 6 servings

Corn Salsa in Avocado Cups

INGREDIENTS
- 1 zucchini, diced
- 2 tablespoons olive oil
- 1 cup fresh or frozen corn kernels
- ½ sweet onion, finely chopped
- 1 tablespoon white balsamic vinegar
- 2 tablespoons minced fresh sage
- 2 Hass avocados, halved and pitted

1. Heat the oil in a large skillet over medium-high heat and sauté the zucchini until it's soft. Reduce heat to medium and add the corn, onion, vinegar, and sage. Continue to cook until the onion is softened, then remove from heat and allow the mixture to cool.

2. Spoon the mixture into the avocado halves and serve.

Makes 4 servings

Broccoli and Garbanzo Bean Salad

INGREDIENTS
- ¼ cup olive or vegetable oil
- 1 clove garlic, minced
- 2 teaspoons unsweetened Dijon mustard
- Salt and freshly ground black pepper, to taste
- 1 can (15 ounces) chickpeas, drained and rinsed
- 2 green onions, chopped
- 1 red bell pepper, chopped
- 2 cups broccoli florets
- ½ cup fresh parsley, chopped

1. In a large bowl, whisk together the oil, minced garlic, mustard, salt, and black pepper.

2. Add the chickpeas, green onions, red bell pepper, and broccoli. Toss so everything is well coated.

3. Cover and place in the refrigerator for at least 2 hours before serving. Gently stir in the parsley just before serving. Keeps well for several days in the refrigerator.

Makes 4 servings

Chickpea Waldorf Salad

INGREDIENTS

Dressing
- ½ cup raw cashews, soaked at least 30 minutes
- Water to cover the cashews
- 1 large clove garlic, minced
- 1 tablespoon fresh lemon juice
- Salt and freshly ground pepper to taste

Salad
- 1 can (15 ounces) chickpeas, drained and rinsed
- 2 ribs celery, finely chopped
- 1 medium-sized apple, finely diced
- 1 cup red grapes, halved lengthwise
- ½ cup diced red onion
- ¼ cup chopped parsley
- ½ cup walnuts, roughly chopped
- 4 cups fresh spinach

1. Make the dressing by first draining and rinsing the soaked cashews. Place the cashews, water, garlic, lemon juice, salt, and pepper in a blender and process until the dressing is smooth. You may need to add more water to reach the correct consistency.

2. In a large bowl, combine the chickpeas, celery, apple, grapes, onion, parsley, and walnuts. Stir in the dressing and toss until evenly coated.

3. Refrigerate for about 30 minutes before serving, or up to 5 days.

4. Serve salad over fresh spinach.

Makes 4 servings

Mango, Avocado, and Black Bean Salad

INGREDIENTS
- 1 can (15 ounces) black beans, drained and rinsed
- 1 red (Spanish) onion, chopped
- 4 Roma tomatoes, chopped
- 1 red bell pepper, chopped
- 1 can (15 ounces) corn kernels, drained
- ⅓ cup roughly chopped cilantro
- 2 Hass avocados, peeled and diced
- 1 mango, peeled and diced
- 4 cups baby spinach

Dressing
- 1 clove garlic, minced
- ½ teaspoon crushed red chili flakes
- 2 tablespoons fresh lime juice
- ¼ cup olive oil

1. Place the beans, onions, tomatoes, pepper, corn, cilantro, avocado, mango, and spinach into the bowl and toss to combine.

2. Place all the dressing ingredients into a small bowl and whisk together until well blended.

3. Dress the salad, adding dressing just until the spinach leaves glisten.

4. Serve. (To prevent wilting of the spinach, dress only the amount of salad you will eat, reserving the remainder for later.)

Makes 8 servings

✓ Orange and Onion Salad

INGREDIENTS
- 2 large oranges, peeled, seeded, and sliced into bite-sized pieces
- 1 small red onion, thinly sliced
- 2 tablespoons rice wine vinegar
- 2 tablespoons unsweetened soy sauce
- 2 teaspoons sesame oil
- ¼ teaspoon grated orange rind
- 3 cups torn red leaf lettuce or baby spinach

1. Arrange the orange and onion in a 13 x 9-inch baking dish and set aside.

2. In a small bowl, whisk together the vinegar, soy sauce, sesame oil, and grated orange rind.

3. Drizzle the vinegar mixture over orange and onion; cover and chill in the refrigerator for at least 30 minutes.

4. To serve, portion the lettuce or baby spinach leaves on individual salad plates. Using a slotted spoon, arrange the orange and onion slices on top of the greens; drizzle the vinegar mixture evenly over salads.

Makes 4 servings

Quinoa Mediterranean Salad

INGREDIENTS
- 1½ cups uncooked quinoa, rinsed and drained
- 3 cups vegetable broth
- 1 large bunch asparagus, stalks cut off and cut into ½-inch pieces
- ½ cup chopped sun-dried tomatoes packed in oil (about 8), plus 2 tablespoons oil (reserved to use in dressing)
- ½ cup pitted Kalamata olives
- ¾ cup red onion, finely chopped
- ¼ cup toasted pine nuts

Dressing
- 1 clove garlic, minced
- 2 tablespoons reserved oil from sun-dried tomatoes
- ¼ cup freshly squeezed lemon juice

- 2 tablespoon fresh oregano, chopped
- 2 tablespoons fresh basil, chopped
- Sea salt and freshly ground black pepper

1. Place the quinoa and the broth in a medium saucepan over medium-high heat and bring to a boil. Reduce the heat to the lowest setting; cover and cook for 15 minutes.

2. Remove the saucepan from the heat and let the mixture stand, covered, for 5 minutes. Fluff the quinoa with a fork and set aside to cool.

3. Steam the asparagus for 2 minutes or until tender-crisp. Transfer to a colander and rinse under ice-cold water to stop the cooking process; drain thoroughly and set aside.

4. In a large bowl, whisk together the dressing ingredients. Add the asparagus, sun-dried tomatoes, olives, onions, and cooled quinoa; toss gently to combine.

5. Serve on individual salad plates topped with toasted pine nuts for garnish.

Makes 8 servings

Quinoa Salad with Black and White Beans

INGREDIENTS
- 1 cup cooked quinoa
- 1 can (15 ounces) black beans, drained and rinsed
- 1 can (15 ounces) white beans, drained and rinsed
- 1 cup diced cucumbers
- ¼ cup diced red onion
- 1 small jalapeño pepper, seeds removed and finely diced
- ¼ cup chopped fresh cilantro

Dressing
- ¼ cup olive oil
- 2 tablespoons fresh lime juice
- 1 tablespoon apple cider vinegar
- 1 clove garlic, minced
- ½ teaspoon chili powder
- 1 teaspoon ground coriander

- ½ teaspoon dried oregano
- ¼ teaspoon salt
- ¼ teaspoon freshly ground black pepper

1. Place the quinoa, black beans, white beans, cucumber, onion, jalapeño pepper, and cilantro in a large bowl; set aside.

2. In a small bowl, whisk together oil, lime juice, vinegar, garlic, chili powder, coriander, oregano, salt, and pepper.

3. Pour the dressing over the salad mixture and gently combine to coat all the ingredients.

Makes 4 servings

Tex-Mex High-Protein Salad

INGREDIENTS
- 2 tablespoons olive oil
- 1 tablespoon fresh lemon juice
- 1 teaspoon cumin
- ¼ teaspoon chili powder
- ¼ teaspoon salt
- 1 can (15 ounces) chickpeas, drained and rinsed
- 1 large tomato, seeded and chopped
- ⅓ cup diced red onion
- 1 Hass avocado, diced
- ¼ cup finely chopped cilantro

1. In a medium bowl, whisk together the oil, lemon juice, cumin, chili powder, and salt.

2. Add the chickpeas, tomatoes, onions, avocado, and cilantro. Toss until combined.

3. Serve immediately for best results. However, the salad can be saved in the refrigerator for up to two days.

Makes 4 servings

Quick and Easy Barley and Lentil Salad

INGREDIENTS
- 1 cup cooked barley
- 1 cup cooked green lentils
- 2 cups fresh cherry or grape tomatoes, halved
- ½ cup finely chopped red onion
- ½ cup chopped cilantro
- ½ fresh lemon, juiced
- 2 tablespoons extra-virgin olive oil
- ½ teaspoon cumin
- Salt and freshly ground black pepper to taste

1. Place all ingredients in a medium-sized serving bowl and gently stir to combine.

2. Season with salt and pepper to taste.

3. Chill for 2 hours to serve cold, or serve at room temperature.

Makes 4 servings

Salad Dressings

Basic Salad Dressing

The essential ratio for vinaigrettes is 3 to 1. As long as you know that, you won't need to consult a recipe every time you want to make a homemade dressing. Just remember 3 parts oil to 1 part vinegar. It's that easy.

One way to keep the two straight is to think about the two ingredients. Oil is smooth and lighter in flavor. Then there's sour vinegar. Can you imagine having a mouthful? That's why you want more of the smooth and light and less of the tangy and mouth-puckering liquid!

INGREDIENTS
- ¾ cup olive oil
- ¼ cup white wine vinegar
- Kosher salt and freshly ground black pepper, to taste

1. Place all the ingredients in a small glass or stainless steel bowl and whisk until fully combined.

2. Let the dressing stand for about 30 minutes to let the flavors meld; whisk the dressing again immediately before serving.

Makes 1 cup of dressing

Basic Vinaigrette

INGREDIENTS
- ¾ cup extra-virgin olive oil
- ¼ cup white wine vinegar
- 2 tablespoons minced green herbs or a pinch of dried herbs (sage, basil, oregano, or your choice)
- Kosher salt and freshly ground black pepper, to taste

1. Place all the ingredients in a glass jar and shake. Or place in a small glass or stainless steel bowl and whisk until fully combined.

2. Let the dressing stand for about 30 minutes to let the flavors meld; whisk the dressing again immediately before serving.

Makes 1 cup of dressing

Mustard Vinaigrette

INGREDIENTS
- ¾ cup extra-virgin olive oil
- ¼ cup white wine vinegar
- ½ teaspoon dry mustard or 1 tablespoon unsweetened Dijon mustard
- Kosher salt and freshly ground black pepper, to taste

1. Place all the ingredients in a glass jar and shake. Or place in a small glass or stainless steel bowl and whisk until fully combined.

2. Let the dressing stand for about 30 minutes to let the flavors meld; whisk the dressing again immediately before serving.

Makes 1 cup of dressing

Vinaigrette for Fruit

INGREDIENTS

Dressing
- 2 teaspoons apple juice
- 1 teaspoon water
- 1 teaspoon rice vinegar
- 1 teaspoon lemon juice
- 1 teaspoon olive oil
- ¼ teaspoon unsweetened Dijon mustard
- ⅛ teaspoon salt

Salad
- Spring mix salad greens
- Assorted fresh fruit, cut into bite-sized pieces

1. Whisk all the dressing ingredients together in a small bowl.

2. Drizzle over greens and fruit.

Makes 1 salad serving with 2 tablespoons of dressing

Dips and Salsas

Asian-Style Dipping Sauce

INGREDIENTS
- 2 tablespoons unsweetened soy sauce or tamari sauce
- 2 tablespoons rice wine vinegar
- ¼ teaspoon toasted sesame oil

1. Whisk together the soy sauce, vinegar, and sesame oil in a small bowl.

2. Serve with sweet potato fries or homemade French fries.

Makes about ½ cup

✓ Basic Salsa

INGREDIENTS
- 2 cups tomatoes, chopped
- 4 cloves garlic, minced
- 1 medium white onion, chopped
- 1–2 jalapeños, finely chopped (adjust to your taste and be sure to use caution, as the jalapeño can cause a burning reaction on hands)
- ¼ cup chopped cilantro, loosely packed
- ¼ teaspoon cumin
- Kosher salt to taste

1. Combine all ingredients in a medium bowl.

2. Cover and refrigerate for one hour. Serve with sliced vegetables or baked chips.

Makes about 2½ cups

✓ Black Bean Hummus

INGREDIENTS
- 1 clove garlic, minced (optional)
- 1 can (15 ounces) black beans, drained (reserve liquid)
- 2 tablespoons fresh lemon juice
- 1–2 tablespoons tahini (sesame paste)
- 1 teaspoon ground cumin
- ½ teaspoon salt
- ¼ teaspoon cayenne pepper

1. Place the garlic, black beans, lemon juice, tahini, cumin, salt, and cayenne pepper into a food processor; process until smooth.

2. One tablespoon at a time, add enough of the reserved liquid from the beans to reach desired consistency, pulsing after each addition.

3. Serve with tortillas or crackers, or as a vegetable dip.

Serves 8

Roasted Red Pepper Dip

INGREDIENTS
- 6 large red bell peppers
- 1 cup golden raisins, coarsely chopped
- ¼ cup plus 2 tablespoons extra-virgin olive oil
- 3 tablespoons salt-packed capers, drained and rinsed well
- 1½ teaspoons coarsely chopped fresh oregano
- Kosher salt
- Red wine vinegar

1. Roast the peppers over a gas flame or under the broiler, turning occasionally, until charred on all sides, about 10 minutes. Transfer to a heatproof bowl and cover with plastic wrap; let stand until cool enough to handle. Peel and seed the peppers.

2. Place the peppers in a food processor and pulse until coarsely chopped. Add the raisins, oil, capers, and oregano; pulse to combine. Season with salt and vinegar to your taste.

3. Serve as a dip with vegetables, baked tortilla chips, or crackers.

Makes 3 cups

Fast and Easy Chickpea Hummus

INGREDIENTS
- One can (15 ounces) chickpeas, drained (reserve the liquid)
- Juice of 1 lemon
- ¼ cup tahini (sesame seed paste)
- 2 tablespoons olive oil
- ½ teaspoon ground cumin
- 1 teaspoon kosher salt, depending on taste

1. Place all the ingredients into your food processor. Pulse to combine ingredients, then blend until smooth.

2. To adjust the thickness of the hummus, add about 1 tablespoon of the reserved chickpea liquid and process for 15 seconds; repeat if necessary to reach desired consistency.

3. Transfer the finished hummus to a bowl and serve. Store your homemade hummus in an airtight container and refrigerate up to one week.

Makes about 1½ cups

Creamy Cashew Dip for Fruit

INGREDIENTS

- ½ cup raw cashews
- ½ cup hot water
- ½ teaspoon ground cinnamon
- Kosher salt to taste
- 2 apples or pears, sliced

1. Soak the cashews in water for 30 minutes. Transfer the water and the cashews to a blender. Add the cinnamon and blend until smooth; season with salt to taste.

2. Serve as a dip with apple or pear slices; or refrigerate in an airtight container for up to 1 week.

Makes 2 servings

Flatbread, Chips, and Crackers

Apple Chips

INGREDIENTS

- 4 apples (crisp apples work best)
- Ground cinnamon

1. Preheat oven to 225 degrees.

2. Wash the apples, then slice crosswise as thinly as possible using a mandoline or very sharp knife to make round slices. Leave the cores in the apples; remove any seeds as you cut.

3. Line baking trays with parchment paper. Lay the apples on the trays in a single layer, as close as possible without touching. Sprinkle with cinnamon.

4. Bake for 1–2 hours, until as crisp as desired. (Bake less time for a chewier chip; baking time also depends on the thickness of the apple slices.)

5. Serve or store in airtight container. You can also chop the slices to use in hot oatmeal.

Makes about 4 servings

✓ Baked Veggie Chips

INGREDIENTS
- 2 medium sweet potatoes
- 2 medium beets
- 2 medium turnips
- Kosher salt
- Olive oil

1. Preheat oven to 275 degrees.

2. Scrub all the vegetables under cool running water.

3. Thinly slice the vegetables using a sharp knife or a mandoline, about 1/16-inch thickness.

4. Lay the slices on paper toweling and sprinkle liberally with kosher salt. Allow to rest for 15–20 minutes, then rinse under cool water and pat dry to remove as much liquid as possible.

5. Line baking sheets with parchment paper and brush with olive oil. Lay the vegetable slices in a single layer on the baking sheets; drizzle the chips with a scant amount of olive oil.

6. Bake in preheated oven for 40–50 minutes, turning the chips about every 15 minutes.

7. Remove from oven, sprinkle with kosher salt, and allow to cool.

8. Serve immediately or store at room temperature in airtight container for up to one week.

Make 6 servings

Butternut Squash Fries

INGREDIENTS
- 1 butternut squash, peeled and cut into french fries
- 4 tablespoons olive oil
- Kosher salt to taste

1. Preheat the oven to 400 degrees.

2. Place the butternut squash french fries in a large bowl and drizzle the olive oil over the wedges. Using your hands, toss the wedges until they are well coated.

3. Line a baking sheet with parchment paper. Arrange the fries so they lie flat on the pan and are not touching each other. Roast for about 25 minutes or until tender.

4. Remove from the oven and sprinkle with the kosher salt; serve.

Makes 4 servings

✓ Kale Chips

INGREDIENTS
- 2 bunches kale
- 2 tablespoons olive oil
- Salt to taste

1. Preheat oven to 300 degrees.

2. Rinse and dry the kale. Remove the leaves from the stems by cutting along the stem with a sharp knife; discard the stems. Cut or tear the leaves to a suitable size for a chip.

3. Place the kale leaves in a large bowl and drizzle with the olive oil.

4. Line two baking trays with parchment paper. Place the kale leaves on the trays in a single layer, spreading them out so the leaves don't touch. Sprinkle with salt.

5. Bake the leaves for about 20 minutes until crisp, watching carefully so they don't burn.

6. Cool slightly before serving or store the chips for several days in an airtight container after cooling completely. Take care when storing, as the chips can break easily.

Makes 4 servings

Homemade Corn Tortillas

Creating your own corn tortillas is easy but may require a little practice. Be sure to save any "mistakes" to bake into homemade chips. Once you've mastered these techniques, it's easy to double this recipe to make more.

INGREDIENTS
- 1 cup masa harina (available in your grocer's Latin foods section)
- ½ teaspoon salt
- ½–¾ cup hot water (from the tap is fine)
- Olive oil

1. Combine the masa harina and the salt in a large bowl. Slowly add the hot water and mix until a dough forms and you can shape it into a ball. Stir with a spatula and then knead the dough a few times with your hands. Form the dough into a ball, cover the bowl with plastic wrap, and let the dough rest for 30–60 minutes.

2. Divide the dough into 8 sections and roll each one into a ball.

3. For the next step, use a tortilla press if you have one. If you don't, cut a plastic zip-top bag around the edges so that you have two matching pieces of plastic. (You can also use parchment paper.) Place one dough ball between the two pieces of plastic; use a rolling pin or apply pressure to a plate to flatten the ball into a circle between 6 and 8 inches in diameter. Slowly peel back one of the pieces of plastic, being careful of the edges, then pull off the other piece of plastic.

4. Brush a little olive oil on the surface of a nonstick pan or a cast-iron skillet; heat over medium-high heat. Place a tortilla in the hot pan and cook for 1 minute; flip and cook the other side for 1 minute.

5. Use for wraps or tacos. You can also cut these into wedges and bake for your own homemade chips.*

Makes 4 servings

* To make chips: Preheat oven to 350 degrees; cut tortillas into wedges and lay flat in a single layer on a baking sheet. Bake for 6 minutes and then turn. Sprinkle with salt and bake for 6–8 more minutes or just until they begin to toast.

Indian Whole Wheat Chapatis

The chapati is a simple flatbread and a staple in Indian kitchens. Making chapatis takes a little practice to master, but once you do, they will become a staple in your home also.

INGREDIENTS
- 2 cups whole wheat flour, plus more for rolling out
- Pinch of fine sea salt
- 1 cup water
- ¼ cup olive oil

1. Blend the flour and salt in a large bowl. While swirling the flour in the bowl with your hand, slowly pour water into the flour until the dough forms into a ball.

2. Either in the bowl or on a counter dusted with flour, gently knead the dough for about 10 minutes. The dough should be soft and pliant.

3. Return the ball of dough to the bowl and brush the surface with a little oil to keep it from drying out. Cover with plastic wrap or a damp cloth and allow the dough to rest for about 30 minutes.

4. When you're ready to fry the chapatis, first assemble your tools: a small, flat bowl of whole wheat flour, a small bowl of olive oil with a small spoon in it, and a paper towel-lined plate or container for the finished flatbreads.

5. Heat a flat griddle or cast-iron skillet over medium-high heat. Meanwhile, on a lightly floured surface, work the ball of dough into a long log. Cut in half, and then in halves again; cut each of the quarters into 3 equal pieces to make 12 equal pieces. Return pieces to the bowl and cover with a damp towel to prevent them from drying out.

6. To form the chapatis, roll a piece of dough between your palms to form a ball, and then flatten with your palm. Place the flattened dough in the bowl of flour; then, using a rolling pin, roll until it's a 4-inch circle. Now spoon about ¼ teaspoon of oil in the center of the circle. Using the back of the spoon, spread out the oil almost to the perimeter of the circle. Fold the circle in half, then in half again, so it forms a triangle. Seal the edges, and dredge in flour again if the dough is sticky.

7. With a rolling pin, start rolling the dough, turning the triangle a quarter-turn after each roll until it's about 6 inches wide with an even thickness. After some practice you'll be able to roll the chapati and rotate it without picking it up.

8. Test the griddle by sprinkling a little flour on it; if it turns brown immediately, it's ready. Gently shake the chapati to remove any excess flour and then place it onto the griddle. It should start browning almost immediately.

9. When small bubbles start to form, spread a little oil over the surface of the chapati and then flip it. The chapati should start to puff up. Spoon a little oil over this side too. When this side of the chapati is puffed up a little more, flip again. Press down on the edges of the flat bread with your spatula to seal the edges and encourage the entire chapati to puff up. If you spot any holes, press down on those too so the air doesn't escape. Allowing the air to stay inside the whole chapati makes it flaky and light.

10. Remove the chapati to your container. Repeat with the remaining dough. Serve the chapatis hot.

Makes about 12 chapatis

Snacks

Roasted Butternut Squash Seeds

When you use butternut squash to make chips, soups, or stews, you'll first remove the seeds. Save them! The seeds are easy to roast and make a pleasant snack.

INGREDIENTS
- Seeds removed from a butternut squash, free of all pulp and rinsed under cold water
- Water
- Olive oil
- Kosher salt

1. Preheat oven to 325 degrees.

2. Bring water to a boil in large saucepan; add salt and the cleaned seeds. Reduce the heat and simmer for 10 minutes.

3. Drain the water from the seeds and pat them dry before transferring them to a bowl. Toss the seeds with olive oil and lightly season with salt.

4. Line a baking tray with parchment paper. Arrange the seeds on the tray in a single layer; roast the seeds in the preheated oven 15–20 minutes. The seeds will not change much in color, but will crunch when done.

5. Store in an airtight container.

Spiced Cashews

INGREDIENTS
- 4 tablespoons apple, orange, or lemon juice
- 4 tablespoons curry powder, cumin, or garam masala
- 1 tablespoon kosher salt
- 3 cups unsalted cashews

1. Preheat oven to 250 degrees. Position racks in the upper and lower thirds of the oven.

2. Whisk together the juice, seasoning, and salt in a large bowl. Add the cashews and gently toss to coat.

3. Line 2 baking sheets with parchment paper. Spread the cashews on the trays in a single layer so they are not touching each other.

4. Place the trays in the preheated oven and bake, stirring every 15 minutes, until dry, about 45 minutes.

5. Cool the nuts completely and then eat or store in an airtight container for up to 3 weeks.

Makes 4 cups

Indian Spiced Pistachio Nuts

INGREDIENTS
- 4 tablespoons apple, orange, or lemon juice
- 4 tablespoons garam masala
- 1 tablespoon kosher salt
- 3 cups unsalted shelled pistachios

1. Preheat oven to 250 degrees. Position racks in the upper and lower thirds of the oven.

2. Whisk together the juice, garam masala, and salt in a large bowl. Add the pistachios and gently toss to coat each of the nuts.

3. Line 2 baking sheets with parchment paper. Spread the pistachios on the trays in a single layer so they are not touching each other.

4. Place the trays in the preheated oven and bake, stirring every 15 minutes, until dry, about 45 minutes.

5. Cool the nuts completely and then eat or store in an airtight container for up to 3 weeks.

Makes 4 cups

✓ Hummus with Cut Vegetables

INGREDIENTS
- 1 recipe of Black Bean Hummus (see page 196)
- 1 red bell pepper
- 1 yellow bell pepper
- 1 pound green beans, steamed and chilled
- 6 carrots, peeled and cut into spears
- 1 cucumber, seeds removed and sliced
- 1 head cauliflower, cored and cut into bite-sized pieces
- 2 large crowns broccoli, cut into bite-sized pieces

1. Arrange sliced vegetables on a serving plate and serve with hummus.

2. Serve immediately and also keep sliced veggies on hand for a quick snack.

Spiced Pecans

INGREDIENTS
- 1 pound pecan halves
- 1½ teaspoons kosher salt
- 1 teaspoon chopped fresh thyme
- 1 teaspoon chopped fresh rosemary
- ½ teaspoon freshly ground pepper
- 1 pinch of cayenne pepper
- 2 tablespoons extra-virgin olive oil

1. Preheat oven to 350 degrees.

2. Spread pecans on a large baking sheet. Roast until fragrant, about 12 minutes. (Watch carefully so they don't burn.)

3. Combine the salt, thyme, rosemary, pepper, and cayenne in a small bowl; set aside.

4. Transfer the roasted pecans to a large bowl. Drizzle with oil and toss well to coat completely. Sprinkle with the spice mixture and toss again.

5. Serve warm or let cool completely and store in an airtight container for up to 2 weeks.

Makes 4 cups

Condiments and Extras

Almond Milk

INGREDIENTS
- 2 cups blanched almonds
- 4 cups water
- 1 teaspoon vanilla extract (optional)

1. Soak almonds overnight and then rinse the nuts until the water runs clear.

2. Place the almonds, 4 cups of fresh water, and the vanilla extract in a blender. Blend for about 90 seconds or until all the almonds are pulverized.

3. Line a fine mesh strainer with a few layers of cheesecloth and strain the blended almond milk, squeezing the milk through the cheesecloth.

4. Refrigerate and use in recipes or on cereal.

Makes 1 quart

Homemade Dijon Mustard

Sometimes it's hard to find prepared unsweetened Dijon mustard. Here is an easy recipe to follow to make your own.

INGREDIENTS
- ¼ cup yellow mustard seeds
- ¼ cup brown mustard seeds
- 1 cup water
- 4 teaspoons mustard powder
- ¼ cup white wine vinegar
- ½ teaspoon sea salt

1. Soak the mustard seeds in the water overnight.

2. Place the seeds and soaking liquid in a blender or food processor along with the mustard powder, vinegar, and sea salt. Process to a paste consistency just like prepared mustard.

3. Transfer to a glass jar for storage. Cover and refrigerate for about 4 days before serving to meld the flavors together well.

Homemade Ketchup

INGREDIENTS
- 2 tablespoons olive oil
- 1 large onion, chopped
- ½ fennel bulb, chopped
- 1 celery rib, chopped
- 1 tablespoon minced or grated fresh gingerroot
- 2 cloves garlic, minced
- 1 large bunch of fresh basil, leaves and chopped stalks
- ½ red chili, seeded and chopped finely

- 1 tablespoon coriander seeds
- 1 teaspoon freshly ground black pepper
- 2 pounds fresh plum tomatoes, chopped
- 1½ cups water
- Scant 1 cup apple cider vinegar
- Sea salt to taste

1. Heat the olive oil in a large saucepan over low heat. Add the onion, fennel, celery, ginger, garlic, basil leaves and chopped stems, chili, coriander seeds, and pepper. Cook for about 12 minutes until the vegetables soften, stirring occasionally.

2. Add the water and the tomatoes to the pot. Simmer gently until the liquid is reduced by half.

3. Place the cooked mixture into a blender and puree, or use an immersion blender in the pot. Strain the sauce through a sieve into a clean saucepan. Add the vinegar and simmer again until the mixture reaches the desired ketchup consistency.

4. Adjust the seasoning to taste with salt; cool in the refrigerator and enjoy.

5. This ketchup recipe can be bottled in sterilized jars and kept for up to 6 months in a cool, dark place.

Quick and Easy Daniel Fast Ketchup

INGREDIENTS
- 1 can (6 ounces) tomato paste
- 2 tablespoons white wine vinegar or lemon juice
- ¼ teaspoon dry mustard
- ⅓ cup water
- ¼ teaspoon cinnamon
- ¼ teaspoon salt
- 1 pinch ground cloves
- 1 pinch ground allspice
- ⅛ teaspoon cayenne pepper, optional

1. Simply combine all the ingredients in a bowl and whisk well to combine. Refrigerate overnight to let the flavors develop, and enjoy!

Makes about ½ cup ketchup

Oatmeal Spice Blend

INGREDIENTS
- 2 teaspoons ground cinnamon
- 2 teaspoons pumpkin pie spice
- ½ teaspoon ground nutmeg
- ½ teaspoon ground cardamom (optional)
- ½ teaspoon ground allspice

1. Place all the spices in a small bowl and blend thoroughly.

2. Transfer to a shaker bottle and use in recipes, or sprinkle on hot oatmeal or fruit.

Makes about ¼ cup seasoning

Twenty-One-Day Daniel Fast Devotional

IN 1 THESSALONIANS 5:23 you can discover an important fact about yourself and how God created you: "Now may the God of peace Himself sanctify you completely; and may your whole *spirit*, *soul*, and *body* be preserved blameless at the coming of our Lord Jesus Christ" (emphasis added).

You are a spirit, you have a soul, and you live in a physical body. Your spirit received new life and was born again when you gave yourself to Christ. Your soul is made up of your emotions, will, intellect, and personality. And your physical body is the flesh and blood of your being. Each part of us needs daily nourishment to stay strong and healthy, and as followers of Jesus Christ, we want every bit of nourishment that comes into us to be aligned with God and His ways.

As you enter into this time of extended prayer and fasting, you will want to begin each day by feeding your spirit through prayer and meeting with the Lord. You can feed your inner person with "soul food," through Christ-centered devotions and teachings, and you will feed your body with nourishing foods and water.

I wrote this series of devotions especially for you as you focus your heart on submitting your whole being to God, with particular attention to offering your body as a living sacrifice. I encourage you to start your day meeting with the Lord and then studying the daily devotion. Begin your day in health and be prepared for the hours ahead. Continue to "check in" with God throughout the day, and allow the Lord to work in your life as you experience the transformation and blessing that awaits you.

DAY ONE

The Temple

> *Do you not know that your body is the temple of the Holy Spirit who is in you, whom you have from God, and you are not your own?*
>
> 1 CORINTHIANS 6:19

First Corinthians 6:19 expresses one of the central concepts behind the Daniel Fast for weight loss. But at first, when we're reminded that our bodies are temples of the Holy Spirit, this truth may stir feelings of guilt or inadequacy. A common response from the soul is, "I know, I know. Jesus died for me! I need to do better. I'll try to do better."

But there is a precious seed of truth in this verse that I

hope will bring you great comfort and encouragement. The truth is that you are not your own. You belong to God. You are His precious child, and He loves you more than you can ever comprehend. His love for you and me is beyond what we can grasp. It's endless love in every direction!

Imagine an earthly father with his precious child nestled in his arms. He tenderly strokes his child's head, and his mind is filled with affection and thanksgiving. As he caresses his young one, he pictures the bright future he wants for this most precious life. He is filled with joy as he imagines the dazzling potential that awaits the child he holds in his arms. He wants the very best for his beloved child, and he will do whatever he can to offer support and encouragement along the way.

Your heavenly Father also wants you to have a bright and hopeful future, and He will be with you all along the way. Hear the words He's whispering into your ear right now: "For I know the thoughts that I think toward you, says the LORD, thoughts of peace and not of evil, to give you a future and a hope" (Jeremiah 29:11).

You are your heavenly Father's precious child. He adores you and He wants the very best for you. You are not all on your own; you are His. And as you enter into this fasting experience, He will be with you. Take hold of His hand, be with Him, and let Him guide you as you walk this part of your journey in faith.

Take Action: Close your eyes. Imagine you are nestled in the arms of God, your loving heavenly Father. Rest in the security of His care. Let Him comfort you. Be still. Be quiet. Receive His love.

DAY TWO

Tending the Tabernacle

> *In the tabernacle of meeting, outside the veil which is before the Testimony, Aaron and his sons shall tend [the lamp] from evening until morning before the LORD. It shall be a statute forever to their generations on behalf of the children of Israel.*
> EXODUS 27:21

Today, as you read these words, your God is asking you to serve Him. He has an important assignment for you, and He hopes you will accept it with honor and dedication. Your Creator is asking you to be the caretaker of His temple, just as He asked Aaron so many thousands of years ago. He wanted Aaron and his descendants to tend to the Tabernacle, to keep it in good order so it could fulfill its God-ordained purpose.

Now He is asking you. Will you tend the temple? Will you take care of your body and give it everything it needs so it can fulfill His purposes? Will you keep it clean and do your best to give it what it needs to stay in good working condition? Will you?

Your Father has a bright future planned for you. He is your biggest fan and your most loyal friend. His promises are sure. His ways are proven. And He is inviting you to accept one of His most worthy posts—to care for His home, His dwelling place.

He doesn't expect you to know everything about how best to care for His home. If you need help, He'll show you the way. If you make a mistake and fall, He'll be there to pick you up, brush you off, and help you continue. He is there for you.

But there is one thing He can't do: make the decision for you. That is your part of the equation. You choose "yes" or "no." You accept the assignment or you don't. One thing you can be sure of is that He hopes you will. He wants you to say yes! You are the only one He's going to ask to fulfill this duty to take care of your body.

Ponder This: Will you accept the call to care for God's dwelling place? What are the key factors in your decision? If you answered yes, what are you willing to do today as you begin this new commitment in your life?

DAY THREE

Love God

You shall love the LORD your God with all your heart, with all your soul, with all your mind, and with all your strength. This is the first commandment.
MARK 12:30

Commandment. It's a heavy word that comes with authority and power. The word means "an important rule given by God that tells people how to behave."

God's commandments are not "pretty please" requests. They are not whims that He hopes you will judge as right and then adopt. No, commandments are hard and fast. They are exactly what our Lord wants us to do. For those of us who see ourselves as His people, His soldiers, His children— they are to be followed. Not questioned, not debated, not changed. Just followed.

God's commandments aren't the kind you expect from most authority figures. He's not telling you to stand up straight and march in a particular cadence. He's not instructing you to clean your room or take out the garbage. He's not ordering you to work extra hours for less pay or holding you to impossible quotas.

No, your Father is commanding you to love Him. Love is the most powerful and the most precious of emotions. When God created you in His image, He planted inside you the ability to love. The Bible says, "We have known and believed the love that God has for us. God is love, and he who abides in love abides in God, and God in him" (1 John 4:16).

As you continue on your days through the Daniel Fast, imagine your heart pouring out more and more love to God. Choose the way of God's heart; choose the way of love. Cast aside anything that will hinder your ability to love God or keep you from falling deeper into a secure and loving relationship with Him. Know for sure that no matter how much you love God, He will always love you more. Oh, what priceless rewards we have available to us!

Meditate: Using your journal or a sheet of paper, write down Mark 12:30. Read the text slowly two or three times, allowing

God's truth to move from your mind into your heart. Now ponder each word and phrase. Make notes about what God is saying to you through His Word.

DAY FOUR

Renewing Your Mind

> *Do not be conformed to this world, but be transformed by the renewing of your mind, that you may prove what is that good and acceptable and perfect will of God.*
> Romans 12:2

As followers of Jesus Christ, we have an invitation from our Creator to live differently. We can decide to follow the teachings of Jesus and then—bit by bit and step by step—turn from the ways of the world and toward the way of the Lord.

The first step for this new and far superior life is making a decision to follow Christ. Next, we begin our quest to change our thinking about how to live. We dig into the Bible and use God's instructions as our manual for life. We study, learn, and gain understanding, and then we begin to change what we think and what we believe to be true.

Renewing our minds from our old ways to the sure ways that align with God is the bridge that leads us to transformation. And transformation is the lasting change that we want. It's the new way of living that brings us the blessing, rest, and joy that Jesus came to give us.

During this time of extended prayer and fasting, you have the opportunity to examine your current way of living and compare it with how God wants you to live from now on. You also can look specifically at how you care for your physical body to discover habits that are not consistent with health and wellness.

These discoveries lead us to actions we can take to change those areas of our lives that are now out of order. We can change the way we think and renew our minds. As we experience renewal about health, eating, and caring for the temple that God has entrusted to us, we become even more fully the new creations in Christ that emerge through transformation.

Fasting Tip: During your time of fasting, pray over each meal and thank God for the good food He designed to nourish your body. Thank Him for the colors, flavors, and goodness present in the vegetables, fruits, whole grains, and other foods He made for the bodies He created.

DAY FIVE

The Operator's Manual

All Scripture is given by inspiration of God, and is profitable for doctrine, for reproof, for correction, for instruction in righteousness, that the man of God may be complete, thoroughly equipped for every good work.
2 TIMOTHY 3:16-17

Before I invited Christ to lead my life, I thought the Bible was just another book. I knew it was popular and included some good teachings, but I thought of it as a book of legends that happened to teach moral lessons. In fact, the Bible was so unimportant to me that when I needed a copy to prepare for a debate, I had to go into my basement and rummage through a box of stored books that I wasn't sure I would ever read.

But then it happened. I started reading the Bible—the Gospels, to be specific—and God's living Word pierced my heart. Waves of truth washed over me, and I knew for sure that the words I was reading were true and that Jesus was real. At that moment my spirit was resuscitated, and I was born again. And I was never the same again!

That was by far the most important change that God's Word has brought into my life. However, over the decades since, His truths have directed my steps and instructed me how to live. Here is one of the most amazing benefits that you and I, as children of God, can have: His holy Word will speak to our spirits and bring about inspiration, motivation, understanding, and change. It's as if we have a backstage pass to access the hidden mysteries of our faith life. As we open our hearts and minds to Him, we receive abundant downloads of truth so our lives can be transformed.

As you study God's Word during your time of prayer and fasting, recognize that the Bible is not "just another book." The Word is alive. Every precept comes from the Most High and Holy God. He has created this instruction manual for us—His people—so we can live the amazing life He has designed for us. That's good news!

Take Action: Write down three of your favorite Scripture verses on individual 3 x 5-inch notecards. Carry them with you throughout the day and periodically read each one prayerfully. Follow with a moment of silence to listen for anything God may be saying to you.

DAY SIX

Present Your Body

> *I beseech you therefore, brethren, by the mercies of God, that you present your bodies a living sacrifice, holy, acceptable to God, which is your reasonable service.*
>
> ROMANS 12:1

Sometimes we read chapters in our Bibles and gain powerful insights. Other times, we can miss or pass over clear instructions. These instructions, when followed, not only bring us into obedience but also deliver freedom, security, and peace.

In this passage, we are being instructed to take a very specific action. The directive is to "present your bodies a living sacrifice" to God. As you let this order seep into your mind, don't be surprised if your heart starts to beat a little faster and you begin to feel slightly anxious. You are being asked to take a profound step. You are being asked to give yourself away . . . as a sacrifice.

From Adam and Eve's first sin to the time of Jesus and His disciples, God's people followed the law of sacrifice. The

Jews were commanded to offer the firstborn of their flocks as sacrifices, and these animals had to be perfect and without blemish. The law was given as a precursor to Jesus Christ, the Firstborn of the Father. Even God gave His Firstborn as a sacrifice so you and I can have eternal life. Jesus offered Himself as a living sacrifice for our sins, and His sacrifice paid for the sins of the whole world.

Today we are being asked to give our bodies as living sacrifices—but not to pay for our sins. Jesus took care of that. Instead, we are called to offer ourselves as living sacrifices in an act of worship and service to our Lord. We are instructed to give ourselves up to God as a humble gift to the One who already has given everything to and for us.

Now we have the choice. Will we let these words just sit on the page, or will we take action? Will we offer ourselves—as people God has already determined to be acceptable—to Him as a living sacrifice? An act of submission? An act of worship?

Action Step and Prayer: Take a few moments to look at your body. Study your hands, your legs, your torso. Think about the truth that your body is not your own. Then use the prayer below to offer yourself as a living sacrifice to the Lord.

Father, at this moment I make the conscious decision to offer this body to You as a living sacrifice, holy and acceptable and to be used for Your service. Amen.

DAY SEVEN

You! God's Creation

God created man in His own image; in the image of
God He created him; male and female He created them.
GENESIS 1:27

God created you in His own image. In the image of God He
created you.

Will you let those words take your breath away? Will you
hold them in your heart as truth and let them penetrate your
thinking? At a time when we are so used to comparing ourselves and our appearance to friends, movie stars, fashion
models, and other "beautiful people," we must let the truth
of who we are shake up our attitude about ourselves. We
must find our peace and security in this fact: God created us
in His own image. Wow! That's amazing.

I've been walking this earth for a long time, and over the
years I've done my share of comparing myself with the image
in my mind of how I wish I looked. I wish my legs were longer. I wish I was prettier. I wish I had a little "less here" and
maybe "a little more there." Thicker hair with more body,
please. And now that I have lived a number of decades, fewer
wrinkles and less sagging would be nice.

But the stabilizing factor in all of this wishing and hoping
is that God made me in His image. He didn't make me in the
Cover Girl image or the *America's Next Top Model* image. No,
He made me in His image, and it's an image that He loves
and cherishes. It's an image that pleases Him.

As I set my mind on the real fact that I am made in the image of God, I sense a stirring inside. It's a shift away from the world's definitions of beauty and a shift toward thankfulness and rest with a sprinkling of awe. I realize, "I am just as God wants me to be."

When I rest in that fact and then use the life of Jesus as my mirror for "how I look today," I will always be just as I was intended to be by the greatest Designer ever. The same goes for you. What a blessing we have when we let the truth govern our lives.

Meditate: Read aloud the words below, inserting yourself into the truth of God's Word:

> God created me in His own image; in the image of God He created me.

Using your journal or a sheet of paper, write down three thoughts provoked by these words. What do they mean for your life?

DAY EIGHT

Wonderfully Made

> *I will praise You, for I am fearfully and wonderfully made; marvelous are Your works, and that my soul knows very well.*
>
> PSALM 139:14

Reading this verse is easy. You might know it well or even have it memorized. That's all good, but now you are invited to go deeper. You are invited to receive this truth into your heart and believe what it says about who you are and what your Creator thinks about you.

When God created you, He did it with intention, purpose, and artistry. He thinks you are marvelous. What a description! *Marvelous* means "causing wonder, astonishing, miraculous, supernatural, or of the highest kind or quality." That's you, dear one! You embody all those attributes.

Do I hear you saying, "Yeah, sure! I see those words, but I don't feel very marvelous"? If so, you are not alone. Most people, deep in their hearts, don't feel great about themselves. That's because we measure our worth and attributes with a faulty measuring tool. We look to the world to tell us if we are good or bad, pretty or handsome, worthy or not. As long as we use the world's standards to measure our worth, we will fall short. We will be making a big mistake.

I hope you will take some time even now and try to put yourself in God's shoes. (I know that's a reach, but go with it for a minute.) Think about Him creating you. Then, like a masterful painter, He steps back and is satisfied with His work. He is full of approval for what He just made. He's almost like an earthly father who sees his precious newborn child for the first time and discovers that his love is greater than he ever knew possible.

Your Creator believes that you are wonderfully made. You are marvelous, one of a kind, precious, valuable. Your Maker is pleased, for you are one of His priceless works.

Praise and Thanksgiving: Spend at least five minutes praising God for making you. Thank Him for His workmanship and the fine details He masterfully created when He fashioned you into His marvelous composition.

DAY NINE

Intricately Fashioned

> *You formed my inward parts; you covered me in*
> *my mother's womb.*
> PSALM 139:13

So often we judge a thing's quality only by its outward appearance. That's natural in today's world of fast glances and quick opinions. But imagine what we miss when we use only the sense of sight to evaluate different objects. Have you ever been served a menu item that didn't look very good, but after just one bite you were convinced that nothing had ever tasted better? Or have you ever watched a video clip of someone in a talent contest? The judges and the audience might have snickered at the contestant's appearance because she looked too old, too young, too plain, or too common. But then the contestant started to release the amazing talent held within her frame, and everyone in the auditorium was astonished.

In a similar way, we often judge our own physical bodies only by what we see on the outside. We mutter and complain about features or traits, and we give little thought to what is actually going on inside of us. Did you know that every three or four days you get a new stomach lining? If you didn't, the strong acids your stomach uses to digest food would also digest your stomach itself. Did you know that your nose can remember more than 50,000 scents?

Did you know that if you took your small intestine and stretched it out straight, it would be about four times as long as you are tall? Think about that! Now look down at your tummy and imagine how God fashioned you so your intestine would fit in that relatively small compartment. And since we're stretching things out, consider your blood vessels. If all the vessels in your body were laid end-to-end, they would measure about 60,000 miles long. You could wrap them around the earth more than two times! Your heart pumps more than 2,000 gallons of blood through those veins every single day.

Every single cell in our body has a purpose, and all the organs work together to perform complex tasks and functions. God designed us that way! Our part is to take good care of what our Creator has constructed. That's what you are doing right now and can continue to do as you stay on your personal journey toward health and wellness.

Ponder: Think about your "inward parts" and the essential functions they perform each minute so that you can live and breathe. Think about your heart, lungs, muscles, and digestive system—all intricately made by the Creator. Given all of that, how do you want to care for this fine masterpiece?

DAY TEN

Choose Life

I call heaven and earth as witnesses today against you, that I have set before you life and death, blessing and cursing; therefore choose life, that both you and your descendants may live.

DEUTERONOMY 30:19

Compare God's command to choose with the common idea that "everything happens for a reason." In many places in the Bible, God tells us that we have options. He lays the choices before us, but then He tells us the best options and the great benefits we can have if we follow His instructions.

On the other hand, when people say, "Well, everything happens for a reason," it often seems like a cover for their own poor decisions. The implication is that our circumstances or the consequences of our actions are all the works of a higher power, and they are meant for our good, no matter what we did to cause them. The problem is that this thinking isn't in line with the Bible.

While of course our all-powerful God is able to bring good out of any circumstance (see Romans 8:28), we are not passive participants. God says we have a choice. In fact, we have choices about many things concerning our faith. The Scriptures are clear about the choice every person has about eternal life. John 3:18 says, "He who believes in Him [the Son of God] is not condemned; but he who does not believe is condemned already, because he has not believed in the name of the only begotten Son of God." We have a choice about what we will believe. God's desire is that everyone will choose the way of Jesus, but the reality is that not everyone will.

In Deuteronomy 30:19, our God is giving us a choice about how to live. We can make choices that will be life-giving or choices that will bring us harm. We can follow His ways or we can choose our own. The decision is ours. And when we choose His ways, we are also choosing Him and His assistance.

Now, over these twenty-one days of fasting, you are presented with choices about how you will care for your body. You are given choices about what you will believe. You are offered choices about how you will eat now and after the fast is over. The good news is that we don't have to guess the right choice. It's easy. It's an open-book test. We only need to say, "Yes, Lord"—and then allow Him to support and guide us as we move forward with Him.

Take Action: What three choices will you act on today that are aligned with God's Word and are life-giving to you and those you love? Prayerfully write them on a piece of paper or in your journal. At the end of the day, check in with yourself and see how you did.

DAY ELEVEN

Don't Defile Yourself

Daniel purposed in his heart that he would not defile himself with the portion of the king's delicacies, nor with the wine which he drank; therefore he requested of the chief of the eunuchs that he might not defile himself.
DANIEL 1:8

One morning when I was on a retreat in Mexico, I took an early morning walk on the beach to talk with God. The scene was breathtakingly beautiful. The sky was blue, with only a few white billowing clouds near the horizon. The sand was soft under my bare feet, and the ocean water was a lovely aqua color. The waves lapped onto the beach in their timely manner. I felt surrounded by our Creator's incomparable artistry.

A gathering of large boulders jutted out into the surf, so I climbed onto one. It served as a perfect perch to take in God's majestic creation as I continued my conversation with Him. Oh, such a lovely morning.

As I sat on the rock, I looked down at the waves splashing among the boulders. That's when I saw the disruption—the out-of-place item that contaminated the perfection of God's masterful work. It was a plastic juice container that someone had tossed away, probably not thinking about how it would mar the excellence that our God has created.

The waves jostled the plastic bottle out of my reach, into crevices where it seemed crabs belonged. Not garbage. Not waste.

As I sat thinking about the scene, I reflected on God's intricate workmanship, including the human body. I thought, *This must be like what happens when the body is working in fine form, and then we put unhealthy foods, chemicals, or highly processed sugar into our systems.* What was working in its ideal way now must cope with the intrusion and make do. Just like the beach didn't choose to have the plastic bottle enter its system, neither do our bodies choose what we give them. Those choices are up to us.

I was thankful that there wasn't more garbage around, at least that I could see. As my walk continued, I picked up three pieces of garbage I found in the sand. This simple beach walk served as a reminder for me to be a good caretaker of the creation God has placed in my charge. I want to give my body what it needs to grow, be nourished, and function in the way my Creator intended.

Ponder: If your body was an ocean beach, what would it look like? Would it be beautiful and pristine? Or would it be more like a dumping ground with lots of contaminants and garbage? During your Daniel Fast, your body is undergoing a major "clean-up." The beach will soon be clean and ready for how you will treat it when the fast is complete.

DAY TWELVE

Enter into Thankfulness

Enter into His gates with thanksgiving, and into His courts with praise. Be thankful to Him, and bless His name. For the LORD is good; His mercy is everlasting, and His truth endures to all generations.

PSALM 100:4-5

I sometimes wonder: If there was a measuring device to calculate how full Christians are of God, would we be close to full, or would we be nearing empty? Would our spirits be healthy and strong, or would we be weak and malnourished?

These seem like good questions to ask ourselves. Am I spiritually strong? Or am I weak and needy?

If it's the latter, there is one sure way to start filling up that empty place in our souls. When we begin to praise God and remember the many blessings He has given us, a change starts taking place in our hearts. The cares seem to dissipate, and the joy of the Lord starts to stir inside. Peace comes to our souls and hope enters our thoughts.

I have had times when I was feeling kind of down. I can stay in that negative place, or I can choose another way: I can turn my attention to my God and begin praising Him and thanking Him for all the good He brings into my life. Before I know it, my heart is flooded with sweet spiritual waves of God's peace. It's almost like an embrace from my Father, who loves me and wants me to look to Him and not my problems. He reminds me to give my cares to Him and to walk according to His ways. Then I will be in His peace, His grace, and His care.

Enter into His gates with thanksgiving and praise. That's almost like our "ticket" to a joyride that is always available to us. It's never scary and is always completely secure.

We have the choice. We can stay outside the gates and grumble and complain and whine and cry. I know. I've done that, and I can tell you, it's not a very fun place to be. I make a much better choice when I wash my face, comb my hair, and start counting my blessings and declaring the goodness of the Lord. It's always the better way to go. It's free, it's freeing, and it's always available to you and to me!

Take Action: Using your journal or a sheet of paper, list ten good things in your life and thank God for them. Don't just mouth the words, but instead wholeheartedly thank your Father for the goodness He brings you. When you are finished with your list, note the way you feel and give thanks again for the change in your attitude.

DAY THIRTEEN

A Living Stone

> *Coming to Him as to a living stone, rejected indeed by men, but chosen by God and precious, you also, as living stones, are being built up a spiritual house, a holy priesthood, to offer up spiritual sacrifices acceptable to God through Jesus Christ.*
>
> 1 PETER 2:4-5

Hmm. I never thought of myself as a living stone. How about you? I surely want to consider it now, though, as I see how God thinks of me!

Go deep with this one and read the passage again. God sees you as something solid. Valuable. Full of life. He's chosen you to be part of His building plan. The Creator of everything wants you to be part of His purpose, to be a member of a holy priesthood that serves the Lord and does His work. Plus, He sees you as one who gives Him spiritual sacrifices that He finds acceptable. That means that, through Jesus, your sacrifices are worthy of God and His greatness.

As you sit today and read these words, embrace this truth about who you are. Shake off the ugly lies and messages the world has sent you about your identity. Toss out the poor self-image notes you repeat to yourself over and over again. Believe God's words about you!

You are special. You are valuable. You are needed. You are holy. And you are His.

When we think about God's vision of us, why would we ever want to look anywhere else for assurance, confirmation, or significance? Yes, those "other places" may have a louder voice or more visibility, but they don't have more truth. And the truth truly will set you free.

Today, are you willing to see yourself the way God sees you? Don't answer that too quickly. Consider what you are saying you will do. From today forward you will take on your new identity, like a newly married person takes on a changed position as spouse. You agree to view yourself as a precious and valuable living stone.

Beginning today, you will counter any messages you hear that are not consistent with what God has declared about you. You will start telling yourself who you really are: Precious. Valuable. Chosen. A member of God's holy priesthood. And His!

Prayer: Spend a few minutes thanking Jesus for His amazing sacrifice that allows you to come to the Father boldly—blameless and of great value to Him. Declare that because of Christ you are worthy, and be the child of God you truly were made to be.

DAY FOURTEEN

Rest Is Waiting for You

Come to Me, all you who labor and are heavy laden, and I will give you rest.
MATTHEW 11:28

Sometimes I close my eyes and calm the buzz going off in my busy mind. I try to imagine the Lord speaking directly to me. Here He's saying, "Come to Me, Susan, and I will give you rest."

I repeat the words over and over again in my mind until I get it—until I can really hear and I don't just slough off the words as ones I've heard so many times before. I try to listen to my Lord Jesus speaking just to me. I listen for the invitation He is offering to me. Here He is offering me rest—not sleep, but rest. Oh, it sounds so good.

Can you hear Jesus offering you rest? Can you take a couple of minutes to calm your nerves, stop your busyness, and hear your sweet Lord calling you, "Come to Me, and I will give you rest"?

His offer isn't conditional. He's not asking you to get your act together and then come to Him. He's not telling you to become a little more worthy before you come to Him. He's calling you right now with no requirements. The only thing you need to do is come. This is one of those times when your spiritual life becomes more real and your actions are for no one else. Just for you, and just between you and Jesus.

Maybe you don't know how to come to Him. What does He mean, anyway?

You don't have to have the answer. You can ask Him. Let Him show you. Let Him speak just to you. Stay quiet, stay calm, and patiently listen with your spiritual ears.

Don't push away an answer that might seem a little silly to you. Is He asking you to move to another seat so you can get out of your comfort zone and hear Him better? Is He asking you to remain silent and open your heart to the peace He wants you to experience as you sit in His presence? Is He asking you to stop worrying and start asking Him for help?

Your Lord Jesus wants you to come to Him. He wants to give you His rest—a rest like no one else can offer you. But before you can have the rest, you must accept His invitation: "Come to Me, and I will give you rest."

Take Action: Sit with Jesus for a while. If being with Jesus in this way is new to you, you may need to practice a few times. Sometimes there are layers of unbelief or self-induced reluctance that need to be removed. Keep at it. Open your heart and your mind, and hear the words of Jesus calling to you. Listen to His words spoken just to you, His precious and much loved friend.

DAY FIFTEEN

Let Him Show the Way

Take My yoke upon you and learn from Me, for I am gentle and lowly in heart, and you will find rest for your souls. For My yoke is easy and My burden is light.
MATTHEW 11:29-30

A yoke is a bar or frame that is attached to the necks of two work animals (such as oxen) so that they can pull a plow or heavy load together. For me, the definition shows even more powerfully what Jesus offers us in these verses from Matthew.

Jesus is calling us to join Him—to put on the frame that holds us together—so He can help us pull the load of life. In case you're picturing yourself like an ox, remember what our Lord says about being yoked with Him. He is gentle and lowly in heart. I like to imagine Jesus' yoke like His arm wrapped around my shoulders so He can guide me through my life journey. That's a comforting picture.

When you put yourself under Jesus' yoke, you are submitting to Him. You are putting your trust in Him and agreeing to walk the way He's walking. And Jesus always walks according to the Holy Spirit. The Bible teaches us, "Walk in the Spirit, and you shall not fulfill the lust of the flesh" (Galatians 5:16). As long as we stay under the yoke and attached to Jesus, we will be walking in the Spirit too. As soon as we slip out from under His covering and care, we are back to our own devices of the flesh. We've walked away from His power, His help, and His protection, and we're on our own.

A yoke is designed for two—in this case, you and Jesus. He's not saying He will take on *your* yoke. Rather, He has a yoke. He has a way. He knows the right direction and the best way to live. His yoke isn't heavy. It's especially designed to come alongside you and fit perfectly on your shoulders so you can walk with confidence, security, and ease.

Here is the really great news: You don't have to walk alone. Jesus is always there for you. He's offering to be right next to you and to lead you as you move into your future. Slip under His yoke. Gladly submit to His direction. Let Him lead you, guide you, and help you pull the load.

Prayer and Thanksgiving: As you enter your last week on your Daniel Fast for Weight Loss, think about the road that's ahead of you. Thank God for what you have learned and experienced. You're free of the controlling cravings and you've taken responsibility for your body's care and well-being. You're almost ready to move into your future with new tools and habits that will support your desire to be healthy.

DAY SIXTEEN

Family Ties

> *Jesus and the ones he makes holy have the same Father.*
> *That is why Jesus is not ashamed to call them his*
> *brothers and sisters.*
>
> HEBREWS 2:11, NLT

Jesus is so much greater than we are that we always feel below Him in might and in stature. No argument there. But there's this little thing about Him and about us: He sees you and me as His siblings! He is not ashamed of us, even though He is so much greater than we are. He still sees us beside Him and with Him.

The reason Jesus can be our brother is because of what He did for us. Jesus made us holy and acceptable to His Father, so we are God's children and part of His family. Your sibling position doesn't kick in far into the future or when you get to heaven. *Today* Jesus is your brother. *Today* God is your Father. And *today* you are a member of the household of faith.

What if we've missed a huge right-here-and-now life-changing truth? What if we've tried to fit this fact about our identity into the world's system and consequently missed out on the blessings we are entitled to because of our birthright? Are we so set in our "I have to see it to believe it" frame of mind that we don't even meditate on this part of God's Word? We just pass the words by until we can sink our teeth into something easier to comprehend. But as a result, we stay low, stay defeated, stay plain and simple and needy.

I know for sure that's not what God wants us to do with this reality about our identity. After all, Hebrews 2:11 says that because Jesus made us holy, we have the same Father. It seems to me that we need to stop passing by these words. We need to spend some time with this truth so that it's not just an idea but something we really believe.

Jesus is our big brother! That is amazingly awesome. First John 3:1 tells us, "Behold what manner of love the Father has bestowed on us, that we should be called children of God!" Today, rest in the knowledge that you are part of God's family.

Meditate: Will you let this truth from God's Word sink into your heart? Don't brush aside the powerful reality of who you are, what you have, and what you can do. You are royalty because Jesus is King and you have close family ties. Get used to it! Wear it. Live it. And be grateful.

DAY SEVENTEEN

Walk in the Spirit

Walk in the Spirit, and you shall not fulfill the lust of the flesh.
GALATIANS 5:16

Robert Frost was the first poet to ignite a spark in my heart. It was because of his "The Road Not Taken" that as a teenage girl I starting thinking about the choices I had and where they would lead me. Even after so many decades, his words still move me:

> *I shall be telling this with a sigh*
> *Somewhere ages and ages hence:*
> *Two roads diverged in a wood, and I—*
> *I took the one less traveled by,*
> *And that has made all the difference.*[1]

Many years later, when I gave my life to Christ and started following Him, I came across Paul's teaching about making a choice between two roads. We can walk by way of the Spirit, or we can walk by way of the flesh. And yes, one is less traveled, but it makes all the difference in our lives.

Every day you and I make choices. We choose how and what we will eat. We decide how to use our time, how to treat people, how to spend our money, and how to lead our lives. Today, our God is showing us that after we first make the decision to walk with Him in the Spirit and follow His ways, all our subsequent decisions will lead us where we really want to go.

It's our choice. We can walk according to God's truth and the directions we learn in His Word, or we can follow the ways of the world and our own plans.

Here is the reality: Our choices set us on a course and then lead to certain consequences. We are the ones who decide which road we will turn to. We are the ones who decide to walk forward, to take a detour, or to stop. The choice is ours and the consequences are ours. Let us choose the right way that leads to life.

Prayer: Today, declare to God your choice to travel the road less taken—to walk in the Spirit and follow the ways of our Lord. You know His way is always the right way. Thank God that He will lead you beside still waters where life is good and you are in His will.

DAY EIGHTEEN

Getting Aligned

Whom the LORD loves He corrects, just as a father the son in whom he delights.
PROVERBS 3:12

You've probably made a lot of mistakes when it comes to taking care of the temple God has entrusted to your care. So have I. But praise God for the good He's doing in us, the new lessons we're learning, and the new habits we're developing.

Your Lord loves you, and that's why you may have felt corrected a few times over the last couple of weeks. I hope you receive His correction as an act of His love toward you. I also hope you respond to His prompts with eagerness to do better rather than with feelings of shame or guilt. Instead, you can thank your Father for His guidance and His calls for you to change and improve your life.

Years ago, I learned a way to help me become more positive

about making mistakes and then changing. I call it "The Next Time." When I do something that doesn't turn out the way I want, or even if I make a blatant mistake, I ask myself, "How will you do it the next time?" This personal query allows me to consider what I've done not so well so I can keep my eyes on the future and plan to be better.

If you find yourself downing a bag of chips or a carton of ice cream, you'll feel discomfort and disappointment. Don't just stay in that negative place without looking for how you can correct the problem. Not considering your actions actually paves the way for more of the same unwanted behavior. Instead, ask yourself, "What will I do next time?" Immediately you will find your mind replaying the thought processes and actions that led you to overeating. When you look at how you can make wiser plans for the next time, you'll practice grace and make a plan. It's like rehearsing the improved version of what just happened.

"Next time I'll put a few chips in a bowl and eat them slowly and enjoy the flavors. Then I'll quit." Or "I'll drink a tall glass of water when I first feel the cravings. I'll pray and ask the Lord to help me. I'll wait to do anything for ten to fifteen minutes and then see if I still want the ice cream."

We all need correction, and our Father corrects us only in love. If you feel any kind of chastisement or shame, it's not from Him. When you do sense His loving encouragement to change, then receive it as His gift for His precious child. He wants only good for you, and He delights in you always.

Take Action: Using your journal or a sheet of paper, write down three weak moments you've experienced related to food and eating choices. Then make a plan for what you will do "the next time" you are faced with the temptations. Imagine yourself making the wise choice and experiencing the victory you want.

DAY NINETEEN

People or God?

Obviously, I'm not trying to win the approval of people, but of God. If pleasing people were my goal, I would not be Christ's servant.

GALATIANS 1:10, NLT

We might need to plaster this Scripture all over our homes so we read it often, let it soak into our understanding, and then really get it! Until we change the way we think, we will try to win the approval of people. It's the way of the world. While some of us struggle with this more than others, we all grow up trying to please people.

This verse shows us how God wants us to live: as "God pleasers" and not as people pleasers. When we live life in this order, all is well. Of course, that doesn't mean we don't care about others. In fact, we please God when we love people and show them respect. We please God when we are kind and considerate. Those are all godly ways for us to treat every person we encounter.

We win God's approval not by being good or walking the straight and narrow. Instead, we please Him when we walk in faith, when we love Him and trust Him, and yes, when we obey Him. Jesus said, "He who has My commandments and keeps them, it is he who loves Me. And he who loves Me will be loved by My Father, and I will love him and manifest Myself to him" (John 14:21). Jesus wants us to follow His ways because that's the best way for us to live.

Today, we can make a life-changing decision to no longer seek the approval of people and instead do what Jesus says to do: "'You shall love the LORD your God with all your heart, with all your soul, and with all your mind.' . . . And . . . 'you shall love your neighbor as yourself'" (Matthew 22:37-39).

Please God. Love people. That's pretty clear. And when we get these truths deeply rooted in our hearts and understanding, we not only will be free from people's judgments of us, but we also will be free to love others more fully and honestly.

Take Action: Make a decision to intentionally love those whom you encounter today. Love them with the love of God that's in your heart. Be the love of God to those who don't yet know Him. In doing this, you will please God.

DAY TWENTY

Day by Day

*We do not lose heart. Even though our outer nature
is wasting away, our inner nature is being renewed
day by day.*

2 CORINTHIANS 4:16, NRSV

We are approaching the end of the Daniel Fast for Weight
Loss, but that doesn't mean our transformation experience is
over. Instead, we are moving into a whole new way of being.
It's a sure and strong way as we embrace the changes that are
going on inside of us. Now that we've had our jump start
using the Daniel Fast, we are ready to begin our journey into
a lifestyle of health.

Your outer nature is changing. Your physical body is getting healthier. You are shedding unwanted pounds. Bit by
bit and step by step, your body is changing. The greatest
change and the most important difference, though, is what
is happening in your heart and mind—your inner nature.

Today's Scripture notes that we do not lose heart. That
means we don't get discouraged, we don't lose hope, and we
don't give up. But there is an action we must include in our
lives for this to be true for us, and it comes at the end of the
verse: "day by day." Our inner nature needs nourishment
each day if it is to stay strong and energetic. We need our
inner nature to be renewed and aligned with God's truth
because it drives our decisions about how we will behave.

I can look back on the many times when I have made

poor choices about my health, about how I react to a situation, or even about how I treat myself or someone else. In every instance, the mistake was because my inner nature was hungry and weak.

The truth is, our mistakes start long before they become actions. The mistake is when we don't invest the time and resources into keeping our inner nature—our spirit and soul—healthy and well-fed on God's truth. We get too busy, we get distracted, or we get lazy. Nourish your inner nature with the Bread of Life each morning.

Ponder: I hope you will make a wise decision to keep the most important part of you—your unique spirit and soul—nourished each day. We know that our physical body needs to be nourished every day. It is even more critical to feed our soul with the rich and wholesome food from God and His Word. What will you do each day to feed your inner nature?

DAY TWENTY-ONE

All for God

Whether you eat or drink, or whatever you do,
do all to the glory of God.
1 CORINTHIANS 10:31

Living for God. That's your goal. It's simple and clear, yet not always easy.

The challenge of living for God isn't on His side of the equation; it's on ours. Lifetime habits and attitudes can be hard to change. However, when we have a deeply established "why" for ourselves—an established purpose for our lives—then moving through change is something we want rather than something we resist.

At the core of why I live my life as I do is that I want to bring glory to God. I want Him to smile every time He thinks of me. I long to hear my Lord say to me, "Well done, good and faithful servant." When I quiet myself and think deeply about my one true "why" for my existence, it always comes down to the same thing: to bring glory to my Father.

My guess is that you also have a big "why" that's your reason for being. Maybe you haven't thought about it or sifted it down to the most important reason for your life, but that "why" is there. I expect that it's close to, if not identical to, mine.

The problem so many Christians have is that we lose sight of our "why." We get so caught up in the details of daily life or the technology of the world, which is constantly clamoring for our attention, that our purpose gets buried. A buried purpose doesn't receive the focus and attention it needs to keep pulling us toward its outcome, so it isn't realized. When we quiet ourselves and think, however, our purpose is still there. It's still the most important reason we have to pursue who God created us to be.

What's the remedy for a buried purpose? To start, we each want to be mindful of our "why"—the reason for our existence. If you wonder about yours, prayerfully consider what God is whispering to you when you pray and study His Word. Peel away all the extra layers of responsibilities and labels and get down to the one true "why are you here?" reason for being.

Once you discover that, ask yourself another question: "What do I need to do to fulfill my 'why'?" The answer may not be just one thing. You will likely have several basic calls to action before you fulfill your "why."

For me, part of bringing glory to God is using the gifts of communication He's given me to share His truths on the platform He's provided. For you, bringing glory to God may also include doing the work He's led you to perform. Perhaps it includes a lay ministry effort, or being involved socially or with family. The uncluttered truth about every follower of Jesus Christ is that we are called to bring glory to God. So as we finish our Daniel Fast and prepare to move into our transformed lives, let's get our "why" unburied and go for it!

Ponder: Take a few minutes to quiet yourself and think about your "why." Consider your purpose and how you can use the special gifts that God has given you to fulfill His desires for your life.

Acknowledgments

My life is richly blessed through the love, generosity, care, and closeness of friends throughout the world. I am better because of you and forever thankful for you. Your friendship nourishes my soul, and your wisdom, intellect, and commitment to excellence inspire me to keep growing. Thank you for your love and support as my traveling companions on this journey called life.

Notes

CHAPTER 2: GET READY

1. "Caffeine Withdrawal Recognized as a Disorder," Johns Hopkins Medicine, accessed April 29, 2015, http://www.hopkinsmedicine.org/press_releases/2004/09_29_04.html.
2. Ibid.

CHAPTER 4: YOUR BODY IMAGE AND WHO YOU ARE IN CHRIST

1. "Anywhere the Eye Can See, It's Likely to See an Ad," *New York Times*, accessed April 29, 2015, http://www.nytimes.com/2007/01/15/business/media/15everywhere.html?_r=0.
2. "Two in Three 13-Year-Old Girls Afraid of Gaining Weight," University of Bristol, Avon Longitudinal Study of Parents and Children, accessed April 29, 2015, http://www.bristol.ac.uk/alspac/news/2013/201.html.
3. "Get the Facts on Eating Disorders," National Eating Disorders Association, accessed April 29, 2015, https://www.nationaleatingdisorders.org/get-facts-eating-disorders.

CHAPTER 5: RESETTING YOUR BODY FOR WEIGHT LOSS AND HEALTH

1. "Profiling Food Consumption in America," *Agriculture Fact Book*, United States Department of Agriculture, accessed April 29, 2015, http://www.usda.gov/factbook/chapter2.pdf.
2. Alice G. Walton, "How Much Sugar Are Americans Eating?" *Forbes*, accessed April 29, 2015, http://www.forbes.com/sites/alicegwalton/2012/08/30/how-much-sugar-are-americans-eating-infographic/.

3. Lindsay Hutton, "Are We Too Sweet? Our Kids' Addiction to Sugar," Family Education, accessed May 19, 2015, http://life.familyeducation.com/nutritional-information/obesity/64270.html

4. "How Well Do You Know Sugar?" The Sugar Association, accessed April 29, 2015, http://www.sugar.org/images/docs/how-well-do-you-know-sugar.pdf.

5. Jeanne Yacoubou, "Is Your Sugar Vegan?" The Vegetarian Resource Group, *Vegetarian Journal* 4 (2007), accessed April 30, 2015, https://www.vrg.org/journal/vj2007issue4/2007_issue4_sugar.php.

6. "Recognizing Added Sugar," Mayo Clinic, accessed April 29, 2015, http://www.mayoclinic.org/healthy-lifestyle/nutrition-and-healthy-eating/in-depth/added-sugar/art-20045328?pg=2.

7. "Chronic Dehydration More Common Than You Think," CBS Miami, July 2, 2013, accessed April 29, 2015, http://miami.cbslocal.com/2013/07/02/chronic-dehydration-more-common-than-you-think/.

8. Ibid.

CHAPTER 7: TEN HABITS FOR HEALTHY LIVING

1. Susan Kelley, "Study: Just a Bite Satisfies Cravings for Snacks," Cornell University, January 30, 2013, accessed April 29, 2015, http://www.news.cornell.edu/stories/2013/01/study-just-bite-satisfies-cravings-snacks.

TWENTY-ONE-DAY DANIEL FAST DEVOTIONAL

1. Robert Frost, "The Road Not Taken," lines 16–20.

Index to Daniel Fast Recipes
for Weight Loss

About the Author

Susan Gregory, "the Daniel Fast Blogger," launched *The Daniel Fast* blog and website in December 2007. Since then, her site has received millions of hits. Susan is passionate to see individuals experience a successful Daniel Fast as they seek God and endeavor to grow in the love and knowledge of Christ. Author of *Out of the Rat Race*, *The Daniel Fast*, and *The Daniel Cure*, Susan has written for nationally known ministries, and her work has taken her to more than thirty-five countries. A mother and grandmother, she lives on a small farm in Washington State.

Visit her online at www.Daniel-Fast.com.

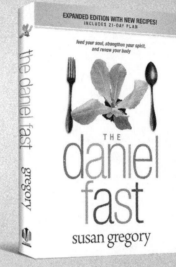
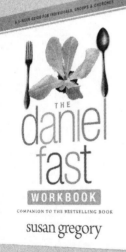

The Daniel Cure

The Daniel Fast Way to Vibrant Health

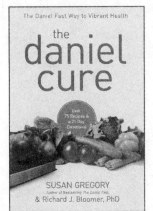

Susan Gregory, Author of Bestselling
The Daniel Fast, *and Richard J. Bloomer*

Though most people begin the Daniel Fast for a spiritual purpose, many are amazed by the physical transformation that takes place, such as a drop in cholesterol, healthy weight loss, a sense of well-being, and increased energy. Recently published scientific studies of the Daniel Fast documented many of the same findings, as well as a reduction in systemic inflammation and blood pressure, and improved antioxidant defenses. *The Daniel Cure* helps readers take the next step by focusing on the health benefits of the Daniel Fast. Following the advice in this book, readers will convert the Daniel Fast from a once-a-year spiritual discipline into a new way of life.

Includes a 21-Day Daniel Cure Devotional, frequently asked questions, ten chapters of recipes, a recipe index, and an appendix detailing "The Science behind the Daniel Fast."

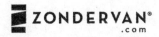
ZONDERVAN®
.com

CP0705